Heal Yourself!
How to Harness Placebo Power

by Beverly A. Potter, Ph.D.
Mark J. Estren, Ph.D.

Ronin Publishing
Berkeley California

Heal Yourself!

How to Harness Placebo Power

Heal Yourself!

How to Harness Placebo Power

Copyright 2013: Beverly A. Potter & Mark J. Estren
ISBN: 978-1-57951-173-9

Published by

Ronin Publishing, Inc.
PO Box 3008
Oakland, CA 94609
www.roninpub.com

Production:

Cover & Book Design: Beverly A. Potter.
Editor: Mark J. Estren.

Cover image: © lina0486 - Fotolia.com

Library of Congress Card Number: 2013922497
Distributed to the book trade by PGW/Perseus

Felix qui potuit rerum cognoscere causas.
                                        —Virgil

Happy is he who can discover the causes of things.

Fere libenter homines id quod volunt credunt.
                                        —Julius Caesar

Men usually believe what they wish to believe.

Other Books by Docpotter

Overcoming Job Burnout:
How To Renew Enthusiasm For Work

Finding A Path With A Heart:
How To Go From Burnout To Bliss

The Worrywart's Companion:
21 Ways to Soothe Yourself And Worry Smart

From Conflict To Cooperation:
How To Mediate A Dispute

Get Peak Performance Every Day:
How to Manage Like a Coach

High Performance Goal Setting:
Using Intuition to Conceive & Achieve Your Dreams

Brain Boosters:
Foods & Drugs That Make You Smarter

Drug Testing At Work:
A Guide For Employers And Employees

The Way Of The Ronin:
Riding The Waves Of Change At Work

Turning Around:
Keys To Motivation And Productivity

Preventing Job Burnout:
A Workbook

Youth Extension A-Z

Beyond Consciousness:
What Happens After Death

Patriots Handbook

Spiritual Secrets for Playing the Game of Life

Simple Pleasures

Question Authority to Think for Yourself

Managing Yourself for Excellence
How to Become a Can-Do Person

Healing Hormones
How to Turn On Natural Chemical to Reduce Stress

Table of Contents

Other Books by Dr. Mark J. Estren

A History of Underground Comics

Statins
Miraculous or Misguided?

Prescription Drug Abuse

Healing Hormones:
How to Turn On Natural Chemicals
to Reduce Stress

Introduction

HEALING MEANS MAKING WHOLE. It is the process of restoring health—becoming whole again. Healing is both physical and psychological—the two cannot be separated. Healing involves repair of tissue, of organs, and of systems, returning them to normal functioning. Healing is a process during which cells regenerate.

How does healing work? What causes it? Is a doctor required for healing to take place? Doctors manage the healing process, deciding upon a strategy, prodding us along—but no, doctors don't heal. Do we need drugs to heal? Again, no—drugs may facilitate healing, but they don't actually "heal." Only the body can heal itself. Perhaps drugs reduce inflammation, or suppress bacterial growth, which helps the body to heal. It is the same with setting a broken bone or suturing a wound. The damaged limb is immobilized so the body can regrow bone, or the skin is sewn together so that it can grow closed—that is, so your living cells can grow and heal the wound.

*Only **living** cells heal you.*

The important thing is that healing occurs in *living* cells and *living* organisms. There is only one thing that can heal your body and that is your living body—you! Every time you've gotten sick and then gotten better, *you* did the healing—you healed yourself in every single case.

How bodies actually heal is a mystery. Healing can be facilitated with a drug or other medical treatment, but the fact is that the body heals itself. Some cancers go into remission—sometimes with no "medical" intervention—while others metastasize. *Heal Yourself* explores ways to start the healing process and to accelerate it by enlisting the power of what scientists call "the placebo effect" to keep ourselves healthy, alert, and full of vigor, so that we can live a good life.

Remembered Wellness

DR. HERBERT BENSON, a professor of medicine in the Harvard Medical School, spent decades researching the mysteries of healing. From the title of Benson's book, *Timeless Healing: The Power and Biology of Belief,* we can tell that psychology—our belief system—plays a powerful role in healing. We must *believe* we will heal. What is the nature of that belief and how does it lead to healing? We will explore this penetrating question throughout this book.

Benson says that the key to healing is what he calls "remembered wellness." His contention is that your body remembers being well, seeks wellness and moves naturally towards wellness. It can be likened to how plants respond to the sun. Plants turn their leaves towards the sunshine and will grow additional branches on the side facing the sun, while the dark side will have fewer branches and leaves. The process is called phototropism—turning towards the light. By turning towards the light, the plant captures maximum energy from the sun, which it converts into life-sustaining energy.

You can observe this yourself by simply placing a leafy plant at a window in your home. The plant can get natural light from only one direction—through the window. Over time, you will actually see its leaves turn toward the window—toward the light. When they have all turned that way, you can rotate the entire plant 180 degrees—and over time, the leaves will turn again, once more seeking the light. Like a doctor with a patient, you are involved in the plant's health—but you are not giving it what it needs to thrive, even if you water it and spray it to ward off bugs. The plant must have light to thrive, and given the right conditions (including water and, if necessary, bug spray), it will seek health-giving sunlight on its own by turning its leaves toward it.

Similarly, each and every cell in your body has what we call a "health-tropic" process wherein the cells "remember wellness" or tend towards healing. All cells in your body move naturally towards wellness or health. But various

All cells in your body move naturally towards wellness.

substances, conditions, and activities, such as stress hormones and foods that are converted into fats, and bad habits—like getting too little sleep—affect cells throughout the body in ways that can lead to imbalance and breakdown.

The trick of healing yourself is to trigger the health-tropic process—in your cells—because healing takes place at the cellular level. The good news is that we know many things about how to harness the mystery of healing, even though we don't understand how it actually works.

Placebo Effect

REMEMBER THAT THE HEALING to which Benson refers occurs physically and psychologically. An area of medical research that has advanced understanding of healing is the *placebo effect*. The placebo effect has been observed in medical research for many decades. It occurs when a drug or other treatment is given to one group to be tested, while a second group that is matched in relevant factors—the control group—receives an inert placebo, such as a sugar pill.

What doctors discovered is that about thirty percent of people who get the fake drug actually improve—and no one can explain how this happens. For a long time, medical research discredited this "magical" healing process by saying "Oh, that's *just* the placebo effect." That didn't explain anything, just dismissed it. But the nagging question remained: how do people who do not get the treatment get better?

More recently, doctors, including Benson and others, began studying the placebo effect and soon realized that it is an important phenomenon: Placebo—the word means "I will please"—holds clues to the mystery of healing. The placebo effect clearly demonstrates that drugs do not heal, that the body does the healing—but how? How can we enlist this powerful process to heal ourselves? How can we turn on this mysterious healing effect? What and where is the switch?

Believe and Expect

THE PLACEBO EFFECT is turned on or off by the beliefs and expectations of the patient—and the healer. When patients *believe* that the drug or treatment will help, it can heal; by contrast, if the drug or treatment is *believed* to be harmful, it can cause negative effects—and even kill. This reverse process is known as the "nocebo effect"—also named from Latin, *nocebo* means "I shall harm." As we shall see in a later chapter, this "expectancy effect" can be enhanced by certain factors, such as the credibility and enthusiasm—or pessimism—of the healer.

Research has shown that the placebo effect can operate on pain, on motor functioning, and on fever, all of which can be directly modified and controlled through biofeedback and other brain training. The body controls the immune system, the sympathetic and parasympathetic nervous systems, and you can enlist them to make yourself well.

When Benson talks about remembered wellness, he is talking about the health-tropic mechanism—your body's innate ability to heal itself. Benson says three components of remembered wellness determine its power. They are:

- First, the belief and expectancy on the part of the patient. Believing you will improve seems to promote improvement.

- Second, the belief and expectancy on the part of the caretaker or doctor.

- Third, the belief and expectancy generated by the relationship *between* the patient and the caretaker.

Belief and expectation are the levers that can turn on— or off—the placebo effect to heal ourselves.

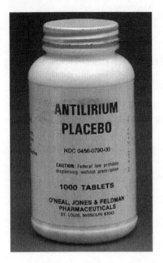

Placebo is not a magic wand. Even though it is mysterious and doctors and scientists don't understand it, we do know many things about the placebo effect. It doesn't work on everything or for every person—certainly not with all people. Researcher Henry Beecher suggested that the placebo effect occurs in about thirty percent of people in control groups.

The placebo effect affects some conditions more strongly than others. It has a particularly strong impact upon pain, swelling, depression and anxiety. It reduces pain in two ways. One is by initiating the release of endorphins, which are natural pain killers created by the brain, and the second is by changing the patient's perception of pain so that it doesn't feel as painful!!

There is something about belief and expectation, especially with regard to our health and our interaction with our healers, that can promote or impede healing. The fascinating thing is that belief and expectation are like levers or triggers that we can turn on—or off—to promote healing.

In the following chapters, we will explore how the brain works, how cells function and communicate, the mysteries of the placebo effect, and how we can harness it to heal ourselves.

2

Power of Placebo

YOU MAY HAVE HEARD THE THEORY that 90 percent of all illnesses are caused by the mind. If so, what are the implications? If most illnesses are caused by the mind, it is likely that most illnesses can be *reversed* by the mind, too.

It is often observed in medical research that people who have gotten the sugar pill and not the medicine in a clinical study get better. This phenomenon is called "the placebo effect." What doctors discovered was that about 30% of people who get the fake treatment actually improve, and no one can explain how this happens. What this means is that for those subjects, their bodies were healed without medical treatment. Those subjects healed themselves.

We revere doctors so much that, even without realizing it, we've developed a belief that doctors and medicines heal bodies. They don't. Only one thing heals you and that's your living body—you. Doctors and medicines facilitate healing, perhaps by reducing swelling or inhibiting infection, for example, but only the body can "heal" the body. That's because healing involves regeneration—production of new, healthy cells and systems.

Spontaneous remission, also called spontaneous healing or spontaneous regression, is more evidence that the body heals itself. Spontaneous healing is an unexpected improvement or cure from a disease. Medical professionals call it "remission," probably out of reluctance to accept that the body has an innate capacity to heal itself. Spontaneous remissions happen frequently and support the notion that the body can heal it self.

Harnessing Healing Power

WE CAN ALTER OUR BODIES by changing our minds. If you were to spend just one or two minutes thinking about someone who wronged you, you would probably start to get angry—or depressed, perhaps—and would feel the impact of those emotions. With anger, for example, you might notice increased heartbeat, tension in your jaw, squinting of your eyes and so forth. If you were to often think about how you've been wronged and victimized, physiological changes that accompany anger would occur like those mentioned plus productuin of stress hormones including corti-sol, adrenaline and norepinephrine, and chemicals such as bile would be released. Over time, being doused with stress hormones can lead to cellular and system dysfunction—breakdown and disease. You can make yourself sick when your mind dwells on unhealthy thoughts!

The placebo effect shows that something that happens solely in the mind can alleviate dysfunction in the body.

The reverse is also true. Whereas unhealthy thoughts can translate into disease, healthy thoughts help the body repair itself. Doctors can facilitate the healing process—but not because of the treatment. It is because of the authority we give them. Supportive doctors help us to "be-lieve" we will get better. As we shall see, belief is central to harnessing the placebo effect for self-healing.

Fake treatments such as sugar pills, saline injections and sham surgeries are routinely used in clinical trials to determine whether a particular drug, surgery or treatment is truly effective.

The term placebo comes from Latin for "I shall please." When we talk about the placebo effect, we're referring to a whole host of events that happen when we bring people into a clinical setting,

The body is a self-healing organism.

give them a treatment that they know may be a genuine treatment or may be a placebo—and pay attention to them. Some patients experience symptom relief and manifest physiological changes from the placebo. Believing that they would feel differently leads them to actually improve.

Positive belief may not be the only factor contributing to the body's response. The body is a self-healing organism, constantly striving to return to a state of balance, known as homeostasis. The body is alive and knows how to regenerate—to heal itself. Our challenge is figuring out how to turn on the healing process.

Belief

THE KEY TO MAKING THIS WORK is *belief.* People who believe that they will get better because the doctor is helping them tend to get better—whether or not the doctor actually gives them real medicine. Many times, doctors do not even know whether they are giving people helpful medicines! In researcheze this is called "double blind," which means that neither the patients nor the doctors know who is getting medicine and who is getting sugar pills, distilled water or something else that has no known effect.

Way back in the 1920s, a doctor cured 88% of people who suffered from a certain kind of wart—and 44% who suffered from a different kind—simply by suggestion: he told them he was going to cure them and they cured themselves.

A few years later, another doctor gave 105 patients the medicine that was commonly used at the time to treat warts—and gave 120 people ordinary distilled water, colored to look like the medicine. This was one of those double-blind experiments in which no one knew who was getting which potion. And you know what? Among patients who got the medicine, 52.5% got better. But in those who got the distilled water, 47.6% got better—almost as many!

This doesn't only work for warts! It can work for serious, even usually fatal diseases. Many doctors have observed that in some patients who are considered beyond treatment, and who get no treatment at all, cancer and other diseases simply go away! A few doctors have looked into this sort of spontaneous remission, thereby contributing to the emerging science of mind-body healing. But most just can't fit what happens with placebo into their medical belief systems. Probably the most common evidence for spontaneous healing is the medically documented case report on a single patient. For example, a patient undergoes exploratory surgery for cancer and the surgeon finds widespread disease. The patient is sewn up and sent home to die, but returns ten years later, for another medical problem. The new physician reviews the medical record and finds the previous surgical report, along with X-rays and other documentation of cancer. He repeats the diagnostic work-up and can find no current evidence of the cancer.

Spontaneous mind-body healing does not only apply to cancer, but is found in a wide range of diseases, including infections, trauma, diabetes, heart disease, skin disorders, depression and many others. These are examples of the body making itself well—harnessing the placebo effect—whether or not the people with the diseases are aware of what they are doing!

No one knows for sure what people who have spontaneous remission are thinking or doing that leads their cancers and other serious illnesses to disappear. People who have healed themselves usually do not know either. But there are patterns that all of us can follow and that point in similar directions. Some people say they prayed constantly for relief from pain or disappearance of their illness. Some say they visualized themselves as being well. Some imagined healing powers helping them—a white light or some other phenomenon penetrating and permeating their body and dissolving or taking away their illness. Some refused to give in to gloom when doctors told them to go home and get their affairs in order— they made it a point to go places, to travel, to spend more time with loved ones. Some created personalized forms of relaxation. Some decided that they needed to laugh more and started finding everything funny they possibly could. And some said they did nothing different at all—they just went about their lives and ignored diseases that doctors said were supposed to be terminal.

We can learn from this! We can harness these and other methods in our everyday lives to help ourselves recover from all sorts of illnesses. Although you may not know exactly *how* these techniques—prayer, visualization, laughter and the rest—tell your cells to make you well, ypu can still *use* the techniques to harness the placebo effect to promote healing yourself

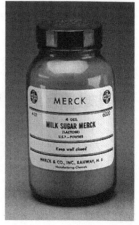

3

Beliefs Rule

BELIEF IS A TYPE OF THOUGHT. It can be a cognition, an attitude, an assumption, or perhaps a theory that emerges from the patterns of electrical impulses in our brain, which we convert into internal dialogue—self-talk, mental images, and emotions. We are largely unaware of these thoughts and feelings as they happen, because the process occurs automatically and non-consciously.

We use the word "non-conscious" rather than unconscious because of the Freudian psychological issues we tend to associate with the unconscious. Non-conscious is used instead to mean outside of consciousness—not conscious.

Belief systems function as "filters" through which we view the world, affecting our physical, psychological and spiritual health. In this filtering process, similarities weigh more heavily than differences. Something is lost, as raw data of the senses become words used to think about what is going on in your world. While these filtered perceptions feel "real," they are *simulations* of events and not the actual events. They come from our talking to ourselves *about* events and their significance.

We live in a simulation created by our beliefs.

Rarely are we aware of this process, so it usually goes unchallenged. Instead we accept our *interpretations* of reality as *being* reality. We respond to what we tell ourselves is out there—our simulations of reality—rather than to reality itself. We live in a simulation, mistaking the words and categories for the events themselves. This goes on so rapidly that it is usually unnoticed.

Checking for Threats

EVEN THOUGH MOST OF US are not aware of it, we are always vigilant and on the alert for threats. Everything is evaluated—appraised—for its potential to bring harm. This goes on rapidly and outside of awareness. Non-consciously we appraise everything: "Am I safe?" "Is this a threat?"

Appraisals are based on past experience and beliefs. An appraisal is a statement of what we expect. The more we encounter certain information, the less we pay attention to it. We give it brief notice, recognizing similarities to previous events, and then make a kneejerk-like prediction about its meaning and significance. This is the appraisal. It is also called categorizing.

We make a rapid appraisal and then put the event into a box or category. You see, we *are* robot-like! We respond to the appraisal—to the simulation, the picture we've created and our beliefs about it—and not to the *actual* event at all.

When the answer is "yes, there is a threat," a second appraisal follows: "Can I stop the threat or get away from it?" Then we respond, not to the situation as it "really" is, but to our appraisal of its threat potential—to our threat simulation.

We See What We Expect

We don't see the world as it is; we see what we believe about the situation.

BECAUSE OF OUR BELIEFS ABOUT A SITU-ATION, our perceptions are filtered so that we overlook valid but contradictory information. As a result of paying less attention to actual sensory data and relying heavily on beliefs about what to expect, appraisals are ultimately based on selectiveperception—because valuable information is blocked out. We simply don't see it because of what we expect to see, even though the information is there to be gathered. We don't see the world as it is; we see what we believe about the situation. This is a simulation.

What this means is that we can change what we "see" by changing our appraisal or analysis of the situation. You may think such things as, "He hurt me." Or, "My boss is out to get me." However, if you slow down the workings of your thinking and closely observe what goes on, you'll probably see that you responded to your appraisal or interpretation of the event rather than the actual event itself.

For example:

> *Event*: My boss said my quarterly report was bad.
>
> *Apprasial*: He was being unfair because he doesn't like me.
>
> *Response*: I'm hurt and I hate this job.

Your response is to your appraisal—not to the event itself. Changing the appraisal would change your response. For example, suppose you looked back at your quarterly report and realized that it was *not* as good as it could have been—perhaps it was disorganized, even though all the good information was in it.

> *Event*: My boss said my quarterly report was bad.
>
> *Apprasial*: He must not have been able to see the information clearly.
>
> *Response*: I need to use a new format and re-submit the report.

Stated another way, your mind gathers the data from its senses, converts them into words and tests them against beliefs, which yields a simulation of what's out there. Then your mind appraises the simulation by asking, "Is there a threat? Yes or no?" Then it responds to the simulation, not the actual event. We respond to our thoughts *about* the situation rather than to the situation itself.

When we believe there is a threat, fight-or-flight is activated and the stress response triggered, flooding us with distress hormones. When this hormonal cascade is triggered by an anxious thought or fear, for example, the hypothalamic pituitary adrenal (HPA) cortical access activates, thereby stimulating the sympathetic nervous system to race in overdrive, pumping up the body's cortisol and adrenaline levels. Over time,

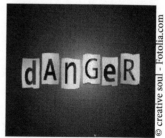

filing the body with these stress hormones can manifest as physical symptoms, predisposing the body to disease. While this process is vital to our survival, it can easily become maladaptive when our beliefs over-estimate or under-estimate threat potential and severity.

Understanding how our beliefs shape our reality is crucial to learning how to heal ourselves, because *belief* that we can do so is a cornerstone of self-healing—of harnessing the placebo response. We have all heard of people who "think themselves sick" by expecting to become ill—and this is a real phenomenon, the opposite of the placebo response. It has its own name: the *noce-bo* response. Many of us remember being told, when we were children, something along the lines of, "Don't be so down-in-the-dumps all

We respond to our thoughts about the situation and not to the situation itself.

the time—you'll make yourself sick!" We all know worry-warts who make themselves sick with worrying. After the 1995 Aum Shinrikyo sarin nerve-gas attack in Tokyo, for example, hospitals were flooded with patients suffering from the highly publicized potential symptoms, like nausea and dizziness, but who had not, it turned out, been exposed to the sarin. This is common in disasters where the agent is invisible, as with chemicals or radiation.

But the opposite is equally valid! "I feel a cold coming on. I'm going to have some warm chicken broth and go to bed early. Tomorrow I *will be* fine!" "Ouch! I twisted my ankle. I'll relax for a few minutes and imagine my ankle as strong and fine and will imagine healing energy rushing to it, and it *will be* fine." These *positive* beliefs are what give the placebo effect its power. Think about it: how many times *have* you had a mild illness or minor injury and gotten better without any medical intervention? For most of us, the answer is, "Many times." We know that, with certain sicknesses or injuries, we can trust our body to heal itself. That is our *belief*—and it is justified and reinforced by experience.

The placebo effect is simply an *extension* of this belief to additional areas and to health issues of greater significance. And just as our belief in self-healing of, say, a minor cut, is reinforced by all the times we *do* self-heal from minor cuts, we can harness placebo with belief that we can heal and will heal.

Expectancy

THERE IS AN ELEMENT of *expectation* that goes with our self-healing. It is important when harnessing the placebo effect. You must believe that you will heal and you must expect to heal. Let's go back to the example of the small cut. Perhaps you put a Band-Aid® on the cut and then forget about it until it heals. You do not think the Band-Aid® *heals* the cut, do you? Of course not—it keeps the cut protected from the elements and from further damage *so your body can heal itself.* After you use this approach for a few small cuts, you *believe* that it will work and you *expect* to get better by keeping the cut covered while your body handles the healing. You *know* that the cut will heal. There is no "if" in your mind.

Similarly, if you take, say, cough medicine for a persistent cough, the medicine does not *heal* the cough—it soothes and calms your throat long enough to allow your body to heal itself. And if this works once, you take cough medicine—very likely the exact same brand—the next time you have a cough, because you *believe* the medicine helps you heal and *expect* that it will do so. If it does not, you are more likely to change brands than to stop using cough medicine altogether—because your belief and expectation are formed by repeated experiences that involve taking medicine and feeling better, and the specific brand...although it may be part of your belief system...matters less than your overall approach to an irritating cough. The cough medicine does not heal you, but becomes part of the ritual of your healing—a facilitation that helps your belief and expectation that you will, indeed, get over your cough.

And so it is with treatments for more-serious conditions. If you *believe* that your body knows how to heal itself and *expect* it to do so, you are paving the way for the placebo response to take control and for your body to make itself feel better. True, it can be more difficult to engage the placebo response when you are dealing with a significant injury or illness, perhaps one that you have never had before—whose treatment is therefore not part of a pattern in your life, as small cuts and coughs are. There is a way to handle this, though—by making your belief and expectation for self-healing explicit rather than implicit. In other words, you can actively tell yourself that you believe your body *can* heal itself (*belief*) and *will* heal itself (*expectation*). The way to do this is by paying attention to your self-talk—as we will see.

4

Desire to Be Well

DO YOU WANT TO BE WELL? The question, posed that way, seems absurd. Of course everyone *wants* to be well! But the answer, from a psychological standpoint, is not so straightforward—and it speaks directly to you being able to harness the placebo effect to heal yourself.

One of Freud's discoveries, many years ago, was that mental illness was difficult to cure because it conferred subtle benefits on people. For example, someone who had a horrific, abusive childhood could have developed ways of coping with it that later, in adulthood, are considered dysfunctional. To handle the constant uncertainty and disorder of his childhood life, he might have become extremely neat and careful in what he did, learning that the only way to keep his parents at bay was to arrange things precisely, keep everything scrupulously clean, and so forth. Internalizing this approach, without even knowing that he was doing so, he could become what we would now call obsessive-compulsive—to such a point that if something in his home is away from its accustomed place, perhaps after his kitchen is cleaned, he becomes intensely anxious, sometimes even physically ill.

We would certainly consider that intense a reaction to a misplaced object to be a form of mental illness—but deep down, the intense reaction is a response to the necessity of self-preservation in childhood, when precision and care provided the only respite from what seemed to him as a child to be terrifying chaos and confusion.

Benefits of Illness

SOME FORMS OF MENTAL ILLNESS do seem to be associated with benefits of certain kinds. Some argue that schizophrenics may have been seen as shamans in ancient societies, and that people with bipolar disorder may be more creative—the condition is especially common among poets. It has also been argued that depressed people are actually more realistic and better able to concentrate on solving problems. As for physical illness, it confers actual benefits in our modern society. The Americans with Disabilities Act guarantees that many people will receive special treatment and accommodation at work, when traveling and as consumers. People with certain physical conditions receive special parking rights, gain easier access to places ranging from stadiums to beaches, get extra attention everywhere from restaurants to gas stations, and get to have pets in "no pet" rental units.

This does not mean that people *want* to be ill, mentally or physically, or that they *want* to stay ill if they have a sickness or disability. Far from it! In fact, chronic illness has disadvantages that are obvious on every level from the personal to the scientific.

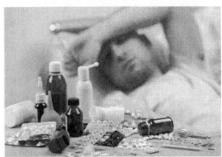
© ia_64 - Fotolia.com

Take those supposed "benefits" of illness, for example. On a simpler, everyday level, someone with the breathing trouble brought on by COPD

or the walking difficulty caused by scoliosis would sure-
ly give up his or her handicapped-parking privileges in
return for an easier and less-painful everyday life.

Still, the notion that there can be benefits to remaining ill is not confined to the realm of psychoanalysis.
How many of us have taken an extra day off from work
at the tail end of a cold or flu, when we are actually well
enough to go back but just feel slightly "under the weather"? In fact, how many of us have used that "under the
weather" feeling, perhaps a mild bit of seasonal affective
disorder or the experience that we *might* be coming down
with a cold, as a reason to stay home and take it easy for
a day? Especially when the weather is cold and unpleasant, the chance to take advantage of being just a little bit
ill can be very rewarding!

And this brings us back to the basic question: *Do you
want to be well?* This is extremely important when considering the placebo effect, be-
cause even though we do not   *Wanting to be cured is*
know precisely how the effect   *an important component*
works or exactly how people   *of harnessing the placebo*
have harnessed it in the past   *effect.*
for relief from illness and even
for spontaneous remission of serious disease, we *do*
know that *wanting* to be cured is an important component of harnessing the placebo effect. It is the foundation
of all the techniques and methods of bringing your body
into the right psychological state so it can heal itself. You
must *want* to be well, *desire* wellness with your whole
heart, in order to put yourself into a state of mind in
which you can try the many possible methods of bringing
the placebo effect into play.

Why do scientists find that, on average, "only" about 30% of people in studies respond when given a placebo rather than a medication or another genuine medical treatment? We have seen that 30% is a remarkable number—and it is! But why *those* people? Why not others? Why not more? There are many reasons, but one of them is certainly *desire*. In clinical trials, people *volunteer* to take part, and clearly those with the strongest desire to be well are the most likely to volunteer. So even people who are not given the genuine medicine are strongly motivated to get better—and with doctors and other health professionals observing them, paying close attention to them and providing far more daily supervision of their care than they usually receive, the people who combine a strong desire for wellness with a strong response to the attentiveness and concern of medical professionals are the ones most likely to benefit from the placebo effect.

Do we *know* this? No. A great deal remains unknown about how the placebo effect works and why it is effective for some people but not others. But there is no question that the *desire* to be well, to recover from whatever illness or condition you may have, is a powerful way to communicate with your body, "telling" it what you want it to do, which is to repair itself. Before trying the many approaches that seem to help the placebo effect take hold, you have to *want* it to work—*want* it to make you well—*want* to feel good. This is the foundation—once you have it there are many ways to build upon it, as we will see.

5

Your Doctor's Attitude

PHYSICIANS PRACTICE SCIENCE, not the healing arts. In fact, the "art" of medicine has waned. But fortunately the word "healing" is beginning to resurface in the practice of medicine. To heal means to make whole. Healing is more commonly heard in alternative medicine and was central in the ancient practice of shamanism. The shaman aided the transformation from illness to health with ceremony and rituals to evoke spirits to diagnose the cause of the illness and to help the person restore balance and wholeness by supporting the patient's belief and expectation of recovery.

Western medicine developed the notion that doctors should be emotionally detached. They should look only at the disease and avoid any emotional interaction that would make diagnosis harder because it was thought that the doctor couldn't be objective—and being "objective" was essential. Modern medicine is a reductionist process of fragmenting a person into organs. It is an expression of the biomedical model of the body as a machine with broken parts. But people are more than the sum of their parts.

Physicians seem to have lost touch with the important role they play as actual people interacting with other people who happen to be patients. Medicine has devolved into a purely intellectual exchange, focused on a physical outcome. Yet healing involves both the physical and the psychological—the emotional, social, and spiritual. Fortunately, doctors are now becoming aware that involving a person—a whole person—is needed for healing.

Many doctors, especially the more traditional ones, are uncomfortable with the placebo response. More and more evidence suggests that something is really going on in this response—and a big part of it is *belief.* When belief is powerful, the placebo response can be dramatic. Shamans and traditional healers knew how to use the power of belief to help their patients heal.

Curing vs. Healing

CURING IS RIDDING THE PATIENT of disease symptoms and the cause of them. *Healing* works to alleviate symptoms by involving the person's psychological, emotional, social and spiritual forces that caused the distress that lead to the illness.

Doctors, nurses, priests and counselors facilitate healing, but they don't cause it. Some of these people have gifts. Some are more open than others. Many things can facilitate healing: petting your dog, gazing at a sunset, sitting under a tree, talking with your friend. Healing is focused on prevention—preventing the disease factors from coming back.

We all know about the bedside manner of the doctor and how important that is, but few doctors do house calls anymore. Patients meet with doctors in medical offices, and offices don't usually have a great ambiance. Physicians could benefit by improving the "feel" of their offices and examining-room environments. They could look at them with a new awareness—with an eye for comforting the patient, such as with engaging pictures on the walls, and having a small water fountain, which gives a soothing sound.

Physicians do have a great deal of power to heal. They also have the power to make the patient get worse, which is the nocebo effect. The doctor-patient relationship has a significant impact on health restoration and maintenance. It is important for doctors to begin to value themselves as healers and to be perceived as healers.

As science progressed, visual proof became the cornerstone in medicine. It is important to the science of medicine to "document" results of treatment—and to be able to replicate those results in multiple people. Obviously a cure that worked only in one person but not in anyone else would do little good. Emotions and the spiritual cannot be seen, so are hard to document, and therefore are considered not to exist—or at least not to be important. More recent research, however, has shown the power of an emotional connection between a patient and doctor is far more likely to led to health improvement during research projects—even when patients are getting the placebo.

What the doctor believes and feels adds to the power of the doctor-patient relationship—remember that in double-blind research, neither doctor nor patient knows whether a drug or placebo is being administered. However, *when the doctor believes* that the patient will improve, the patient is much more likely to do so—even when receiving no real treatment. Anything that a doctor can do to improve the bond with his or her patients, to provide hope and confidence, can potentially translate into huge improvements in the patient.

Doctor As Healer

FIND A DOCTOR YOU CAN TRUST and believe in, who will
help you feel hopeful and inspired. Increasingly, science
is showing that hope heals—maybe not perfectly and
maybe not completely, but hope has a tremendously
powerful healing power. Hope, optimism, a warm connection with the doctor—these are strong medicine even if
they do not guarantee success. In fact, studies show that
people who are very high on perfectionism tend not to be
able to establish positive rela-
tionships with doctors, maybe
because no one can be perfect
enough. Perfectionists seem to
do particularly poorly on ther-
apeutic outcomes of depression—a field in which a lot of
the research was conducted.

*The central skill of a
healer is the capacity to
awaken hope in patients.*

The central skill of a healer is the capacity to awaken
hope in patients and the ability to provide meaningful
explanations of the sickness, allowing people to re-estab-
lish order in their lives. This is what the ancients did.

Desire is a strong motivating force. A strong desire for
healing, no matter how it is felt, is essential for getting
and staying well. Here the concept of *allowing* is important. Allowing is the process of receiving healing—and is
the opposite of striving. Allowing is a process of receiving—surrender is important. One does not surrender to
an illness, but one may surrender to a higher will. And
that is the role that ancient healers played and that some
doctors can play today.

A good doctor-patient relationship maximizes harnessing placebo. Increasingly, doctors are coming to believe that medicine is about treating a person rather than

a disease and that the emotional needs of the patient are vital to recovery. This leads to the conclusion that doctor-patient rituals can have a tremendous positive impact on the patient's healing.

Evidence for the importance of this relationship is mounting. A study conducted at Harvard, using people with irritable bowel syndrome, allegedly examined the effects of acupuncture. Participants either received treatment from a researcher who was warm, caring and engaged them in friendly conversation—or from one who was curt, distant and said little. In each case *there was actually no acupuncture administered.* The treatment was a sham, with fake needles that did not puncture the skin. The results were stunning. Even though there was no acupuncture performed, the patients treated by the caring researcher improved as would be expected if they had been receiving a powerful drug: a whopping 62% actually got better. Conversely, the improvement level of those treated by the less-pleasant researcher was only 28%. This is strong testimony to the power of the placebo effect—and the power of health professionals to engage or fail to engage it.

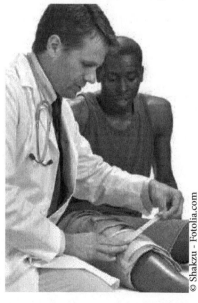

© Shakzu - Fotolia.com

The placebo effect shows the ability of our minds and hearts to heal. While it happens non-consciously—outside of consciousness—it isn't random: healing happens when the conditions are right, when the patient believes in his or her own healing transformation and when belief is reinforced by interaction with a caring person.

The doctor-patient relationship is one of the primary influences on a patient's belief that a treatment will work. When doctors are caring and believe in the work that they are doing, and when they take interest in the patient, they create conditions for healing to happen. When patients feel strongly that they are receiving the treatment they need, they non-consciously tap into whatever it is that we call the placebo effect—which means reaching right down to the cells to stimulate them to work in harmony and to heal.

The patient's belief makes a world of difference as to that person's health. In fact, what a doctor says and what the patient believes may be more closely tied to the patient's outcome than what the doctor does physically. Thus, if a doctor's warnings about possible negative side effects increase the likelihood of the patient experiencing pain or suffering, as research consistently suggests will happen, then the leading culprit is the patient's mental state. Fear or a deep pessimism—an expectation of not getting better—can be the underlying enemy of health.

It is important to realize that while an inert sugar pill (placebo) can make you feel better, warnings of fictional side effects (nocebo) can make you feel those, too. This is a common problem in pharmaceutical trials; for instance, a 1980s study found that heart patients were far more likely to suffer side effects from their blood-thinning medication if they had first been warned of the medication's side-effects.

Should doctors warn patients about side-effects when it might trigger nocebo?

This poses an ethical quandary: should doctors warn patients about side-effects if doing so makes the problems more likely to arise? There is still no definitive answer to that question. Doctors tend to make a decision on a case-by-case basis, although the threat of malpractice lawsuits more often leads them to reveal everything about possible medication problems—thus inadvertently undermining the effectiveness of treatment for at least some patients.

Avoiding Nocebo

THE NOCEBO EFFECT MUST BE WATCHED CAREFULLY by doctors. By monitoring pain levels in volunteers who had been given a strong opioid painkiller, researchers found that telling a study participant that the drug had now worn off was enough for a person's pain to return to the levels it was at before the drug was administered. This indicates that a patient's negative expectations have the power to undermine the effectiveness of a treatment, and suggests that doctors would do well to treat the beliefs of their patients, not just their physical symptoms.

All this research places a spotlight on doctor-patient relationships. Today's society is litigious and skeptical, and if doctors over-emphasize side-effects to their patients to avoid being sued, or patients mistrust their doctor's chosen course of action, the nocebo effect can cause a treatment to fail before it has begun. It also introduces a paradox—we must believe in our doctors if we are to gain the full benefits of their prescribed treatments, but if we trust in them too strongly, we can actually die from their negative pronouncements. For example, researchers found that if a doctor discusses a serious prognosis ("you have six months to live"), the likelihood of a patient dying within that time frame rises. Labeling a patient with a negative prognosis may be robbing him or her of the hope that regaining health may be possible—and this becomes a self-fulfilling prophecy when the patient manifests the decline that the doctor has said to expect.

What all this means is that patients get better in part because they believe in the power and effectiveness of modern medicine and expect a sense of relief after seeing their doctor—they place faith and trust in medical professionals. In fact, a nurturing therapeutic relationship may be in large part what is in operation in engaging the placebo effect. Optimism and trust are important in the relationship between the doctor and the patient, with a large impact on the patient's recovery. What the doctor believes about the patient's prognosis matters: the doctor's expectations influence how the patient responds. Indeed, when a doctor believes a patient is likely to improve, the patient *is* more likely to improve.

Even the personality of the doctor has an impact on healing. When the doctor exudes warmth, attention and confidence, patients are more likely to get better. It may be that the doctor actually triggers the healing response—the doctor becomes the placebo. The exact way this works is unknown, but researchers have some ideas about it. It seems likely that when the patient attributes positive meaning to a doctor's statements and trusts the doctor to take care of him or her, the patient's stress response is minimized and the relaxation response is engaged. The mind is soothed, fear alleviated, and the body relaxes—into a state in which the cells' health-tropic nature comes to the fore and the body stays focused on healing itself. The patient starts to get better right away—powerful testimony to the importance of doctor-patient relationships and the potency of the placebo response.

Is My Doctor a Healer?

READ THE DESCRIPTIONS of doctor activity below. Remembering your last few visits, rate your doctor on a scale of 1 to 5 for each activity, with 1 being "does not do this at all" and 5 being "does this very well."

___ 1.My doctor listens to me.

___ 2. My doctor has an open heart.

___ 3. My doctor looks at me in a comforting way.

___ 4. My doctor sits when talking to me.

___ 5. My doctor is there for me.

___ 6. My doctor has a healing touch.

___ 7. My doctor is a partner in keeping me healthy.

___ 8. My doctor avoids judging me.

___ 9. My doctor explains and teaches.

___ 10. My doctor is optimistic about my health.

___ 11. My doctor trusts my intuition.

___ 12. My doctor respects others who help me.

___ 13. My doctor helps me feel that I belong.

___ 14. My doctor has a relaxing manner.

___ 15. My doctor offers me hope.

Scoring:

15 is the lowest score and 75 is the highest.

15-30: Your doctor may be a good clinician but is low in the warmth and support needed to help you harness the placebo effect. You would be wise to find a new doctor.

31-45 Your doctor shows some signs of warmth, but this is not his or her main quality. Consider looking for a new doctor, unless this one's clinical knowledge and experience is crucial for your condition.

46-60 Your doctor shows considerable warmth and attentiveness to your needs. If he or she also has strong clinical experience, this can be a good match for you, combining scientific knowledge with ability to engage the placebo response.

61-75: Your doctor has strong healer qualities and is likely to combine empathy with strong science knowledge, which is the best combination.

The score is a guide and not an absolute. Use the score to think about qualities of your doctor and to compare doctors you are considereing. The empathy score should always be combined with clinical training and experience.

Find Your Doctor

ASK YOUR FRIENDS and family about their doctors. On-line doctor-rating sites may be helpful. Another place to look is an academic medical center, which is a hospital linked to a medical school, sometimes called a teaching hospital.

Always check out credentials. More important than where docters graduate is the hospital where they do their residency, which is their on-the-job training. Also important is where doctors practice because they are highly influenced by the clinical style of other MDs they practice with. Being Board-Certified and affiliated with a reputable hospital. Is important. Your insurance company's website will generally list credentials and affiliations.

You might call the doctor's office blind. Notice how the phone is answered and how you are greeted. Hoe the receptionist treats you may be a sign of the doctor's style.

Trust Your Gut

ALWAYS TRUST YOUR "GUT" RESPONSE. How do you feel while talking with this doctor? Do you feel comfortable— safe and supported? How empathetic and engaged is the physician? It is helpful to take three or four questions about your health issues with you to your first appointment. As the doctor answers your queries, notice how the doctor explains things, Are you given time to ask follow-up questions? A doctor who makes you feel comfortable and listens to your concerns may be your perfect match.

6

Your Amazing Brain

WHEN YOU HEAR THAT YOU CAN HEAL YOURSELF without drugs, you may wonder if that means that you "decide" or "make up your mind" to heal—that healing yourself is a conscious, "willed" decision. That is not how self-healing works. To engage the placebo effect, you must go *around* consciousness to communicate your desire for healing directly to your cells, because healing takes place at the cellular level.

Consciously deciding to heal would be quite a feat. Only a small amount of what goes on in our brains is consciousness—1/100,000 or so, scientists tell us. That's 0.001% of the time, which mean that 99.999% of what the brain does is not conscious! Most of the time our "thinking" is non-conscious—outside of consciousness.

So how much energy does it take to run the human brain? According to Stanford computer scientist and bioengineering professor Kwabena Boahen, a robot with a processor as smart as the human brain would require at least 10 megawatts to operate. That's the amount of energy produced by a small hydroelectric plant. But our body does not contain any such industrial plant.

You've probably noticed the parallel between the way computers and our brains function. Like computers, our brains use energy to process information. Scientists have determined that even though the brain weighs less than 2% of the body, when at rest it consumes 20% of the body's energy—it uses energy at 10 times the rate of the rest of the body per gram of tissue.

Imagine your brain as a computer hard drive. How much memory would your "system" have? A few scientists have puzzled over this question in recent years, with widely varying results. Syracuse University Professor Robert Birge estimates that the human brain has a storage capacity of between 1 and 10 terabytes. To give a frame of reference, high-end personal computers come with 1 terabyte of memory. Northwestern University psychologist Paul Reber estimates that the brain's memory storage capacity is 2.5 petabytes—which equals 1 million gigabytes, or 1,000 terabytes. The entire print collection of the U.S. Library of Congress is estimated at 10 terabytes. By any measure, our brains are amazing.

The human brain operates on only about 20 watts of continuous power— half the juice needed to run a small light bulb on your back porch!

Surprisingly, according to professor of mechanical engineering Bill Burnett of the Stanford University Design School, the consensus is that the human brain operates on only about 20 watts of continuous power, depending upon its activity. That's half the amount of juice needed to run a small light bulb on your back porch!

By comparison, a desktop computer uses about 175 watts, while a Z3 super-computer uses 4000 watts— and Watson, the legendary computer named after IBM founder Thomas J. Watson, needed 80,000 watts per

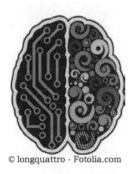
© longquattro - Fotolia.com

hour when answering questions. These high-powered computers can manage unfathomable amounts of information and do complicated statistical calculations in seconds; but, as Burnett points out, computers can't fall in love. They can't write a poem. They can't found and run a company.

Here is another way of looking at this: our brain uses 200 to 400 kilocalories per day, which equates to between 10 and 25 watts of power. For comparison's sake, that's about 10 to 25 percent of the power that it takes to run a 100-watt light bulb. A regular computer performing the same number of calculations the same way the brain does would take more than 40 million times the energy that the brain uses. Extraordinary!

How can the brain accomplish such complicated work at such low energy—less than what the light bulb on the back porch needs? Even more puzzling, how can such a low-wattage brain heal the living human body? The answer, as we shall see, is that much of our "brain power" actually goes on at lower levels, at the cellular level.

Self-Healing

WE CANNOT WAVE A MAGIC WAND like the good witch from *The Wizard of Oz* and command ourselves to be well. Rather, healing takes place somewhere in the non-conscious—somewhere below and outside of consciousness. We understand how we can consciously think, "Stand up," and then actually stand up—or at least we think we understand. It's familiar. But *how* do we command an activity that takes place outside of awareness? What do we *do*? What do we *think*? How do we reach that place? This is the underlying confusion, because healing goes on without thinking, or, more precisely, it goes on *outside of thinking*. This is what mystics mean when they say, "Get out of your mind," which sounds like "go crazy" but actually means "let go of thinking —of talking to yourself."

Our bodies function wonderfully—perfectly, in fact— without our conscious mind directing them. Healing goes on at the cellular level. The challenge is to communicate with our cells. How is this done? And what do we communicate?

Information Overload

IMAGINE THE DISTRACTION if you were consciously determining every action, including breathing, moving blood around, walking, noticing how high to raise your feet, and so forth. It would be paralyzing. We don't need to know about most of the stuff going on in the mind or body, any more than we need to be paying attention to the pistons in the engines of our cars to drive one across town.

"Awareness is a limited capacity system," explains Professor Emanuel Donchin of the University of South Florida's Department of Psychology. "I have no idea how I search memory or get grammatically correct sentences out of my mouth. It's hard enough to handle the little that reaches awareness. We'd be in terrible shape if everything were conscious."

A huge amount of information bombards us continuously, coming in through our eyes, ears, nose, tongue, and skin. Were we to process all of the incoming information consciously, the

We filter out irrelevant data with the use of schemas.

brain certainly could not run on less than the power of a low-wattage light bulb. It would have to be vastly more powerful. But filters in our sensors cut out what's irrelevant according to a set of *schemas.*

Intelligence is found throughout the body—in every cell—and not just in the brain. Cells are not just blobs of tissue; cells are alive, they have intelligence, and they tend towards wellness—health-tropism. Much incoming visual information is pre-processed on the optic nerve path before it gets to the brain. Muscles and nerves have "muscle memory" that calls up schemas to register where your body is in space. Then muscles react to the schema, without any direct conscious processing by the brain. This type of process goes on throughout the body—"non-consciously," that is, outside of consciousness.

What we see when we look out into the world is filtered and sent into a part of the brain that we have no awareness of—the non-conscious.

Schemas Explained

IN *The Psychology of Self-Deception: Vital Lies, Simple Truths*, University of California at San Diego emeritus cognitive psychologist Don Norman argues that we notice and remember what is *relevant*. The judgment of relevancy is orchestrated by schemas—a term psychologists use for the mental files in which we organize and store information. Our experiences are sorted into schemas—and this tremendously reduces demand for conscious brain power, for having to pay attention.

*A **schema** is a cognitive framework or concept that helps organize and interpret information.*

Through the use of schemas, most everyday situations do not require conscious, effortful processing. We quickly organize new perceptions into schemas and act on them without conscious effort—a process also sometimes called "categorizing." In other words, a schema is a cognitive framework or concept that helps organize and interpret information. Schemas are loosely connected by association. They allow us to take shortcuts in interpreting the vast amount of information coming in from our environment, enabling us to make quick judgments and act without much, if any, conscious thinking.

British psychologist Frederic Bartlett introduced the concept of mental schemas as part of his learning theory. In Bartlett's theory, our understanding of the world is formed by a network of abstract mental structures. The result is an intricate dance, as schemas and attention interact. Attention to one facet of experience—"I can hear my chickens clucking and it is morning"—activates relevant schemas, such as thoughts of letting the hens into the yard, throwing out feed, and checking for eggs in the brooding box. The schemas are a little like apps on a smartphone—they guide attention and provide shortcuts to action. When a farmer walks into the yard with the "chicken schema" active, his focus is on the chicken coop, not on the field that needs plowing or on feeding the dogs. Schemas determine the scope of attention. Schemas determine what we will notice; they also determine what we ignore.

We have a schema for everything. We have a schema for dog. A schema for chair, for ice cream cone. We have a schema for faces and a neural path that encodes the face of a teacher, the face of your spouse, your child. It takes considerable processing the first few times we see

someone to recognize that person again. We evolve schemas quickly, so that after not too long we develop neural
paths that encode the information of the new person's
face into a schema for that person.

Non–Conscious to Preconscious

WHEN SOMETHING HAPPENS, we load up and run the appropriate schema—all outside of awareness—non-consciously. When there is a change in the environment, a schema
loads up into our preconscious to run. We think that
consciousness is everything, but we are actually aware
of only about .001% of the processing going on in our
brains. The other 99.999% of the brain is not idle; we're
just *not consciously aware* of its operation. It is only
when we bring something into consciousness that we
become aware of it. Our brains are able to work at a low
energy level because what we are aware of through verbal
and conscious activity is a tiny fraction of the processing
in operation.

How we chunk or schematize information is important. Schemas can get in the way of our health, because
*we don't see what we are looking at—we only see what
we are looking for.* We get stuck in schematic thinking
and only see the possibilities we're seeking. Healing yourself is about expanding those possibilities—developing
new, more health-tropic schemas.

Consciousness

BY STUDYING PEOPLE with brain damage, scientists discovered that the brain is organized into consciousness,
short-term memory and long-term memory. Short-term
memory lasts seven to ten minutes. Consciousness is
only about 300 milliseconds long, which provides about

half a second to grasp and store what we are aware of. Schemas enable us to grasp relevant information from the world in 300-millisecond snippets and put it into short-term memory.

If the information is important and needs to be encoded, it becomes part of long-term memory. Metaphorically, the brain creates a movie, frame by frame, of what we see—and the way we put the movie together is with our schemas. They can also be thought of as "programs." Either way, healing yourself involves creating health-tropic schemas, so your body focuses non-consciously on keeping you well and fighting off disease.

The Preconscious

WE HAVE A PRECONSCIOUS BUFFER in the brain that takes information and makes predictions about what will happen next, and this is how we tie together a consistent notion of our existence—in other words, how we construct reality. Reality is not objective in the sense that the reality is actually "there." If it were, everyone would share the same experiences and the same beliefs about those experiences. Rather, what we regard as reality is what we perceive through our schemas—which are formed through our own unique experiences and therefore differ, sometimes substantially, from the schemas of other people.

If you don't like reality, change your mind.

Biologist Bruce Lipton explains in his book, *The Wisdom of the Cells*, that the conscious mind can process about 40 bits of data per second. That is, it can take 40 different kinds of inputs to juggle per second. The non-conscious mind, which is everywhere in your body because each cell has intelligence and is "thinking" non-consciously—enables it to process 40 million bits of data in the same second. Thus, the non-conscious mind is one million times more powerful as an information processor than the conscious mind. Most of our cognitive activity—95 to 99 percent—goes on in the non-conscious mind; less than five percent of neural activity is influenced or controlled by the conscious mind. Similarly, 95 to 99 percent of our behavior is derived from the perceptions programmed in the non-conscious mind.

We cannot communicate directly with our non-conscious, which is responsible for control of nearly all our autonomic and automatic bodily processes—including what our cells do. But we can construct schemas that will cause our non-conscious to focus on healing us and keeping us well, which is how we engage the placebo effect. The key is finding ways in our conscious mind and behavior to produce schemas that the non-conscious will use in a health-tropic manner.

7

Community of Cells

WHEN YOU LOOK IN A MIRROR, you see yourself as one person—a single entity. While this is a clear observation at the macro level, it is also a misperception. You are actually a community of about 10 trillion living cells *plus* host to another 100 trillion intestinal bacteria that process the fuel to keep those 10 trillion cells going. These are astonishing, nearly inconceivable numbers, and truly astronomical—they are the sorts of numbers we hear when scientists discuss distances to other parts of the universe, not numbers we associate with our own bodies.

Even more remarkably, each cell is a living individual being. Every cell has its own life. Every cell has its own functions. Every cell interacts with other cells in its community. So while you appear to yourself as a singular entity, you are actually a colony organism. If you were reduced to the size of your cells, you'd see a busy metropolis of trillions of individuals living in harmony—when you are

Each cell is a living individual.

healthy. Each of us is a collective consciousness of trillions and trillions of individual cells living in community, functioning in various degrees of harmony or disharmony.

Interestingly, major functions in the human body also occur in every cell. For example, your body has digestive, respiratory, reproductive and waste elimination systems. And the function of each of these systems also exists in every cell of your body—each individual cell consumes nutrients, reproduces, excretes wastes, and breathes.

Furthermore, just as we know how much the environment influences us on a conscious level, so does the cellular environment influence each cell within our body. This makes intuitive sense. Most of us respond positively to bright, sunny weather and mild temperatures—not only physically but also psychologically. We simply feel better when our external environment has a more positive feeling to it. But when the days are dark and cold and the weather compounds the gloom with cold rain, ice or snow, most of us feel physically drained even when we are not actually sick—and emotionally exhausted as well. There is even a condition called Seasonal Affective Disorder to describe a severe level of these symptoms.

The point is that we respond quite directly to the external environment. Sometimes there is a direct threat from outside to which we need to react—in the case of weather, it could be an ice storm or hurricane, for example. But most of the time there is no such threat—just a different composition of elements of the environment, to which we respond in a positive or negative way.

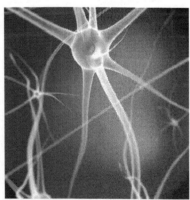

© Giovanni Cancemi - Fotolia.com

The same is true for our cells. *Their* external environment consists of the bodily organs and fluids within which the cells exist. Sometimes there is an external threat—for example, from disease-causing organisms. But most of the time, what determines the cells' environment is an increase or decrease in the body's own production of specific chemicals that have a direct impact on the cells' behavior. The chemicals are produced by your autonomic nervous system at a non-conscious level—but you can learn to affect their production in ways that are favorable to your health.

Brain of the Cell

WE TEND TO THINK THAT THE NUCLEUS, which contains the genes, is the cell's brain. However, that's not the case, at least in the sense of a brain as a control mechanism without which the cell cannot function. The nucleus is in control of the cell's reproductive mechanism. When scientists remove the cell's nucleus, the cell doesn't die. Biologist Bruce Lipton's research has taken a different approach, arguing that the cell's skin or membrane is the cell's "brain" and that it is the functional element that controls the cell's life.

It is the cell membrane that perceives environmental signals and then translates those signals into biological signals that control our life and our body's functions. And this is a key to making ourselves more health-tropic—to encouraging our body to keep us well and restore us to health if anything gets in the way of our preferred state of being, which is wellness.

The cell membrane is important because that is where we can and do change the environment to which our cells respond—and to which, therefore,

It is at the membrane that the cell encounters its environment.

our body as a whole responds. The cells' environment can be filled with chemicals that have positive or negative effects. For example, when we react with stress to an occurrence, our *sympathetic nervous system* causes our body to produce the stress hormones *cortisone, adrenaline* (also called *epinephrine*) and *norepinephrine.* In modern life, when stressful events seem to be never-ending, many of us live in a near-constant state of heightened stress-hormone production. And that means that our cells are constantly bathed in these hormones—which are known to suppress the immune system, thus making us more vulnerable to disease. Therefore, by responding with a stress reaction to events in our lives—which, to put it another way, entails provoking a fight-or-flight response, as if there is physical danger to be dealt with—we are "telling" our cells to get ready for an emergency, which reduces our body's immune response. This allows opportunistic viruses or bacteria in the environment—there are always some around—to more easily get through the cell membranes and begin the process of causing disease.

We communicate with our cells indirectly— non-consciously.

Healthful Environment

CONVERSELY, when we feel calm, when we remind ourselves that the everyday irritations we feel are *not* crises and therefore not worthy of the flood of hormones associated with the fight-or-flight response, we engage the hormones produced by our *parasympathetic nervous system.* This system balances the sympathetic nervous system through the production of hormones associated with calm, restfulness and relaxation, including dopamine, endorphins, serotonin, oxytocin and nitric oxide. A cellular environment rich in these healing hormones is one in which the cells can remain health-tropic, focused on maintaining and strengthening their defenses against potential external threats from viruses, bacteria, even toxic chemicals.

We cannot directly tell our cells to focus on keeping us well and fighting off threats to our health, but we can behave in ways that alter the cells' environment and thus encourage each cell—and our body as a whole—to behave in a health-tropic fashion. This is how we harness the placebo effect.

As humans occupying our human body, we constantly review and perceive the environment, then adjust our biology accordingly. For example, when our skin receptors perceive that it is cold, our blood vessels contract to preserve heat; when our skin receptors sense that it is hot, we sweat to release heat. Not all of our perceptions are accurate, however. While growing up and going through daily life, we acquire perceptions that may be incorrect or skewed in unhealthful directions. Because our bodies convert perceptions into biology, if we are laboring under misperceptions, those misperceptions can lead to maladjustments of our biology—opening us up to physical or psychological illness.

For example, for unknown reasons, some people's immune systems turn against normal cells within the body itself—and send out warrior cells to eradicate them. The result can be diseases as serious and debilitating as type 1 diabetes and rheumatoid arthritis. Some treat-

We can no longer pretend that the patient's perceptions don't matter. And we can't pretend that healing is something doctors do to a patient. Your mind is in every cell of your body.
—David Felten, PhD,
University of Rochester
School of Medicine

ments of autoimmune diseases revolve around getting
the body to recognize that the healthy cells it is attacking
are not in fact enemies—that is, changing the body's
perception of those cells so that, operating at a non-conscious level, it will stop destroying them.

Perceptions control many of our reactions at a conscious level, too. When things are not going well, we need
to change our perceptions—our interpretation of events
in the environment. This is something we can achieve
through mental activities—you can behave in ways that
will make yourself afraid or make yourself calm. To harness the placebo effect, we need to behave *consciously*
in ways that will pervade our body, causing its *non-conscious* processes to produce a cellular environment more
conducive to health and wellness. The good news is that
this is not only possible but also a goal that is attainable
in a number of different ways—so you can try one, several or many of them to find which will be best for you.

8

How We Stress Ourselves

A S INFANTS AND TODDLERS, we are not critical thinkers. We believe what our parents, siblings, teachers, and other adults say. As a child, you may have been told, "What a beautiful little girl." Or "You're no good. You will always fail." "You are strong and healthy." Or, "You will always be sickly and weak. You'll probably get cancer just like your grandfather." Children don't question what they hear about themselves; they believe it as facts. And then, like computer programs, these beliefs or scripts run our lives as we get older.

You've probably noticed that thoughts run through your mind almost all the time. Observing more closely, you'll probably notice that it seems like someone—who?—is talking to you, inside your head. Who is talking to you? You are!! Psychologists call this "self-talk." We repeat over and over to ourselves the things we heard said about us—in a kind of self-indoctrination. When you make a mistake, you may say to yourself, "Dummy! You dummy, you always screw up. You'll never amount to anything. Dummy!!" Our non-conscious minds interpret such negativity as a "threat"—just as if your mother or teacher were saying it. And this triggers the release of stress hormones that affect our cells, our health and our mood.

Starting in childhood, we gather a list of attributes that describes who we are in the world. "I am a teacher, mother, Italian, Democrat, line dancer." And who we are as a person: "I am a klutz with women, I can't learn a foreign language, I am not likable, I will never be successful because I can't handle money." Then we repeat the list to ourselves—again and again, although not consciously—and thus reinforce our self-beliefs. We cement ourselves into the programs that we tell ourselves and that come to define us.

Here is a useful exercise: Take a look at some of the beliefs you hold. Write them down. *Try this now.* Choose something you "know" about yourself. It can be positive, negative or neutral, and can involve any part of your life. Here are some possible examples. "I work better on a team than alone." "I have a strong family orientation." "My faith sustains me." "I can't stop procrastinating." "When I have easy and hard tasks to do, I like to get the easy ones done first."

Then *question* whatever you "know" about yourself. "What makes me sure that I work better as a team member?" "How do I know I cannot stop procrastinating?" If you are like most of us, you will come up with a series of examples that back up your statement—times when you did well on a team, for instance, or times when you procrastinated. *But those examples do not prove what you "know."* They only show you doing things in accordance with what you *think* you know.

Dig deeper. Try to get back to your childhood, where so many of our self-impressions get their start. You may work on corporate teams now—did you always play team sports as a child? Why? Did your parents push you into them? Were you trying to gain acceptance from peers? Were you reluctant to stand out on your own for fear of failure? Did you enjoy the feeling of boosting other people's performance? And how about procrastination? Did you find homework difficult, so you kept putting it off? Did you have games to play and friends to visit, so you simply ignored other matters until you <u>had</u> to deal with them? Did you get a "charge" out of waiting until something was almost due, then rushing to finish it? Did your last-minute work gain you praise for its quality, so you had no reason to work faster or sooner?

The specific reasons for what you "know" do not matter—what matters is that you question what you "know," then decide whether it is really correct. You may decide that it <u>is</u> correct—or maybe not. The important element is the questioning, not the specific answers.

The purpose of this exercise is to figure out *how* you "know" what you "know." Some beliefs are accurate, but many are 100% false. And whether true or false, they can have significant influence on behavior. Here are some examples.

Belief System A

> ***Event:*** A person is lying in the gutter.
>
> ***Appraisal:*** Only bums lie in gutters.
>
> ***Response:*** That person is a bum. I'll cross the street to stay away from him.

Belief System B

> ***Event:*** A person is lying in the gutter.
>
> ***Appraisal:*** Lying in the gutter is not normal.
>
> ***Response:*** That person may need help. I'll go to him and find out.

Belief System A

> *Event:* A snake is in the path.
>
> *Appraisal:* Snakes are dangerous.
>
> *Response:* Fear, panic, screaming, attempt to escape.

Belief System B

> *Event:* A snake is in the path.
>
> *Appraisal:* Snakes are interesting.
>
> *Response:* What luck to see one!

Mind and Body Are Connected

BELIEF SYSTEMS CORRELATE not only with behavior toward those around us but also with how we behave toward ourselves. Research by cellular biologist and author of *The Biology of Belief: Unleashing the Power of Consciousness, Matter and Miracles,* Dr. Bruce Lipton, reveals that our thoughts actually affect the cells in our bodies. *Science Daily* reported that the reviewers of more than one hundred sixty studies on the mind-body connection were shocked by the consistency they saw in the data. Over and over the evidence showed that a person's positive beliefs have a strong influence on his or her health.

Our bodies have two different protection systems. The *immune system* deals with internal threats such as viruses,

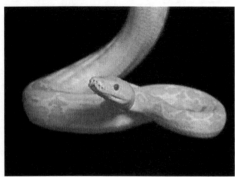
© Alexey Kuznetsov - Fotolia.com

bacteria, parasites or cancer cells. The *adrenal system* responds to external threats, such as a poisonous snake or a mugger, by secreting stress hormones that engage our protective fight-or-flight response. These hormones constrict the blood vessels in the gut, forcing blood to the arms and legs where it nourishes fight-or-flight behavior. Growth and immune functions are inhibited during fight-or-flight in order to ready the body for action.

Everyday stresses trigger fight-or-flight, which re-presses the normal functions of both the growth and immune systems to conserve energy. With enough stress, we reach a point where we do not replace the number of cells we lose, leading to organ and tissue dysfunction—the primary cause of disease. Reduced immune activity also opens us up to attack by normally suppressed in-fectious agents. Stress constricts the flow of blood in the forebrain, sending it instead to nourish the hindbrain's high-speed reflex center, which controls the behavior used in stressful situations. Since the forebrain is where our consciousness and intelligence reside, shutting down its function because of stress causes us to behave less intelligently.

A growing body of research in mind-body medicine demonstrates an undeniable interplay among biomedical, psychological and social factors, and points specifical-ly to a causal link between psychological problems and many physical illnesses. The field of *psychoneuroimmu-nology* is demonstrating that stressful life events can adversely affect the immune system.

For example, researchers found that depression—already known to be caused by heart disease in many patients—can also be a *precursor* of heart disease, with certain depressed patients being fifty percent more likely to develop or die from heart disease than those without such symptoms, even though they had no prior history of heart disease. Depression, therefore, likely affects not only the mind but also physical health—by being linked to increased blood pressure and abnormal heart rhythms, as well as chronically elevated stress hormone levels, which can increase the heart's workload.

It is thought that the mind-body link is mediated by the executive functions of the prefrontal cortex of the brain. Interestingly, placebo responses are disrupted in people with Alzheimer's disease, and this supports the theory that the area of the brain related to belief is damaged in Alzheimer's—with belief being central to the effectiveness of the placebo response, as we have seen.

Most of us don't notice how often we think, that is, talk to ourselves about unhealthiness. We take for granted that the risks, symptoms, aches and pains of health are involuntary. We don't question such thinking; we just do it. Our negative emotions tend to be exacerbated, causing us to feel dread, stressed-out, hostile, hopeless, depressed, debilitated by guilt or shame in situations where concern, frustration, annoyance, sadness or regret would be more appropriate emotions.

There is another, better way. It involves switching our self-talk from a focus on the inevitability of illness, debilitation and decline to a focus on hope. A focus on what builds confidence. On thoughts and conversations about health that counteract fear rather than adding to it. On ways in which an increase in spirituality—compassion, prayer, forgiveness—grounds us in positive expectations and purges negative ones. It is this refocusing, this change in our self-talk in the direction of *belief* in our self-healing abilities and *expectation* that we can make ourselves well, that will engage the placebo effect and in so doing have an ongoing positive impact on our health.

Here are examples of typical negative self-talk statements about health—and more-hopeful ones to which you can switch *without ignoring the underlying realities.* This is important, since recommending a blind belief in optimism is unrealistic and invites even greater disappointment if the placebo response does *not* come into play, or a worrisome health matter *does* come to pass. Do not go from pessimism to blind, Pollyanna optimism—simply accept that negative possibilities exist, *but so do positive ones,* and focus on the pluses rather than the minuses.

Negative:	Hopeful:
My father died of heart failure at 66. I'm 60 and probably have only six years to live.	My father died of heart failure at 66. Because I know that, there are steps I can take to keep my heart strong and take command of my own health—such as exercising more and improving my diet.
The gastroenterologist found polyps during my colonoscopy. That means I'm at high risk for colon cancer.	Thank goodness the doctor found those polyps. Now I can take positive steps to make cancer less likely, such as increasing my daily fiber intake.

My vision keeps getting worse, which at my age probably means cataracts or macular degeneration. Oh no, I'm going blind.	My vision keeps getting worse. I will look into ways to strengthen it—and find out what the options are for preventing it from becoming a serious issue.

In each of these examples, the original observation remains the same—it is a reality of health with which we need to deal. But the *response* to the reality changes, from passive acceptance and "awfulizing" to an understanding that something negative in health does *not* necessarily lead to *further* negatives, and that there are *active* things we can do to prevent an admittedly negative situation from becoming worse. The two words to remember here are *take control.* Negative thinking is a form of giving control up—surrendering to a disease, to family history, to a prognosis, or simply to what a doctor says. The more-hopeful approach involves *taking control* by accepting that negative circumstances exist, but denying that those circumstances *must* lead to additional negatives. Taking control through hopeful self-talk sends your body a message, all the way to the cellular level, that what you want is to be well, to get better, to engage the placebo effect in order to improve your health both now and in the future.

9

Relax

IT IS HELPFUL TO THINK of the human body as a machine—
and it *is* a kind of bio-chemical machine, run by an
amazing computer-like brain. The problem is that while
we may be in the driver's seat of a bio-robot that carries us
through life—we don't know how to drive the thing. Oh, we
can make it move and can get pretty good at doing so. You
might keep it on the road of life, or run it into the ground,
or crash it into a wall. Learning to operate your magnificent
body is largely a trial and error challenge.

There are all kinds of important variables you must take
into consideration when operating your body, like what
food you eat, when and how much. Breathing is another
operational tool—although not one you normally need to
think about. Another tool is thinking, what psychologists
call "self-talk". You know from your own experience that
self-talk, especially about problems and worries, stimulates
anxiety, which triggers the stress response. This is not a
bad thing if you understand your bio-robot well so that
you can purposefully "activate" it, rev it up. It is not a good
thing when your body frequently launches the stress response without your meaning to so that "it is happening *to
you*." That's when things go wrong and the body begins to
malfunction and break down.

Relaxation

THE BEST WAY TO UNDERSTAND the relaxation response
is to look at its opposite, the stress response. The sympathetic nervous system reacts to stress by secreting
hormones that mobilize the body's muscles and organs
to face a threat. Sometimes called the "fight-or-flight
response," this mobilization includes a variety of biological elements, including shifting blood flow from the limbs
to the organs and increased blood pressure. The body
responds to stress by moving into a state of readiness
with an internal secretion of cortisone, epinephrine and
norepinephrine.

The problem is that the stress response is largely
an either or response. Research shows that the body
responds to *change* as a threat. With change there is
always a degree of uncertainty, of risk, which is threatening and kicks in the stress response. This means that the
stress response does not require an emergency; it can be
triggered by everyday worries and pressures.

The body is built to launch into a state of alert readiness for short bursts *only*. When the readiness state
becomes chronic things can—and do—go wrong. This is
what happens in response to ordinary daily worries and
hassles, so that most of us are chronically stressed—
chronically revving our bio-robot. There can be anxiety
from continual adrenaline release, which promotes high
blood pressure and cardiac irregularities, and may lead
to hostility and anger, pain, insomnia, impotence and
other dysfunctions. Our bodies are not built to handle
chronic stress, which leads to breakdown and disease.

You do control your bio-robot. You *can* quickly relax your body with breathing and repetitive thinking. When you focus on your breathing—when repeating a word (or a sentence, a prayer, a sound, a phrase) on the out breath, while passively disregarding thoughts to return to the repetition—you will experience remarkable bodily changes: decreased metabolism, decreased heart rate, decreased rate of breathing, decreased blood pressure, and slower brain waves.

You can purposefully relax your body when you know how. You can purposefully give your heart a rest by slowing your heart rate and reducing your blood pressure, all by slowing your rate of breathing and changing the content of your thoughts.

Health Benefits of Deep Relaxation

RELAXATION DOES LOTS OF GOOD THINGS for your body. The benefits of practicing a relaxation technique are overwhelming. Regular practice of relaxation techniques will assist you in relieving muscle tension, reducing anxiety, and improving your overall well-being.

Increased Immunity

DEEP RELAXATION, if practiced regularly, can strengthen the immune system and produce a host of other medically valuable physiological changes. Relaxation boosts immunity in recovering cancer patients. An Ohio State University study found that daily practice of progressive muscular relaxation significantly reduced breast-cancer recurrence. Another study showed that a month of relaxation exercises boosted natural killer cells in the elderly, giving them a greater resistance to viruses and tumors.

Lower Blood Pressure

A HARVARD MEDICAL SCHOOL STUDY found that meditation lowered blood pressure by making the body less responsive to stress hormones, similar to effects from blood-pressure-lowering medication. Several studies have shown that patients trained in how to relax had significantly lower blood pressure.

Dr. Herbert Benson of Harvard Medical School found that regular sessions of simple meditation decreased the body's response to norepinephrine, a stress hormone. "Ordinarily, norepinephrine stimulates the cardiovascular system," Dr. Benson said. "But regular relaxation training resulted in less blood pressure increase from norepinephrine than is usually seen. Relaxation shows results similar to the action of the beta-blocking drugs used to control blood pressure." Moreover, the research shows, relaxation may help ward off disease by making people less susceptible to viruses, and by lowering blood pressure and cholesterol levels.

Reduces inflammation

INFLAMMATION IS LINKED to heart disease, arthritis, asthma, and skin conditions such as psoriasis. Emory University researchers say stress is the villain. Relaxation switches off the stress response.

Asthma

RELAXATION WIDENS restricted respiratory passages, so it can offer relief to asthmatics by diminishing the emotional upsets that trigger attacks and the constriction of air passages that closes breathing, according to a report from Rutgers Medical School. The effects were most pronounced for those who suffer chronic asthma, rather than seasonal.

Pain

A MAJOR BOON OF RELAXATION TRAINING is in alleviating chronic, severe pain, including backache and chronic migraine or tension headaches, and pain from diseases such as cancer. Dr. Benson says that for many of his patients, the relaxation response can be evoked by their sitting quietly with eyes closed for 15 minutes twice daily, and mentally repeating a simple word or sound. "Eighty percent of patients choose a simple prayer to repeat," Dr. Benson said.

Stress

RELAXATION IS AN IMPORTANT TOOL in reducing daily stress. Just a few minutes of deep relaxation is an effective way to refresh your mind and body, offering increased energy levels that lead to balance and healing. When performed regularly, relaxation exercises can have noticeable effects on your stress levels and mood.

Self-Observation

GIVEN ALL THE BENEFITS OF RELAXATION, it makes sense for all of us to learn how to do it. The relaxation response is a way of "telling" our body, down to the cellular level, that there are no imminent threats and no reason to rev up for fight or flight—but there *is* reason to stay calm and balanced, to allow the cells to engage in their usual health-tropic activities without having to face some sort of dangerous external change.

We have all felt the tension in our muscles when we are under stress or feeling upset. To relax effectively, we need to know how to get rid of that tension, replacing it with its opposite.

The first step is to learn to discriminate between sensations of tension and those of relaxation. Try this now. *Lightly* tense your left hand to make a fist. Tense just enough to notice the tension. Objectively and dispassionately notice exactly where and how the sensation of tension feels. Next, deliberately create contrast in the sensations by *quickly* releasing the tension and consciously relaxing the muscles in your left hand, while objectively watching what you experience. In a detached manner, compare how your hand feels when relaxed with how it felt when tense.

Learning to identify tension in your muscles involves systematically tensing and relaxing various muscle groups throughout your body, one at a time, while studying how the sensations feel in the muscle when tense and when relaxed, as you did in the tense-fist experiment. The objective is to learn to identify small amounts of tension so that you can then take action to reduce the tension *before* it gets to an extreme—so that you can bring your activation level back into the optimal range.

Study Tension to Relax

FIND A PLACE where you can be comfortable and won't be disturbed for about a half hour. Lie on your bed, couch,

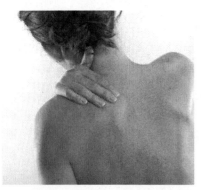

or a futon on the floor, or alternatively sit in an over-stuffed chair. Kick off your shoes and loosen your belt and any tight clothing.

Tense and relax each muscle in the list of muscle groups below, one at a time, as follows. With eyes closed, tighten the muscle just enough to notice the tension, as you did with the fist experiment. It is important to learn to detect light tension, so *do not tense tightly*. While holding the tension for about seven seconds (except for the feet—hold these for three seconds), study the physical sensation of tension in the muscle.

Next, *quickly release* the tension from the muscle, relaxing it as much as you can, while studying the sensation of relaxation for ten or more seconds. Compare the sensations of relaxation and tension. Then tighten the muscle just enough to notice the tension a second time, while studying how and where the tension feels for you. Compare the feeling of tension to the feeling of relaxation. Then *quickly release* the tension and relax the muscle as much as you can. Study the way relaxation feels and compare that feeling to the way that the tension felt.

Muscle Groups

Arms and Hands

Hand and forearm: Make a fist.

Biceps: Bend the arm at the elbow and make a "he-man" muscle.

Face and Throat

Face: Squint your eyes, wrinkle your nose, and try to pull your whole face into a point at the center.

Forehead: Knit or raise eyebrows.

Cheeks: While clenching your teeth, pull the corners of your mouth toward your ears.

Nose and upper lip: With your mouth slightly open, slowly bring your upper lip down to your lower lip.

Mouth: Bring your lips together into a tight point, then press your lips into your teeth. Blow out gently to relax.

Lips and tongue: With your teeth slightly apart, press your lips together and push your tongue into the top of your mouth.

Chin: With your arms crossed over your chest, stick out your chin and turn it slowly as far as it will go to the left. Repeat for the right side.

Neck: Push your chin into your chest at the same time as pushing your head backward into the back of your chair to create a counter force.

Upper Body

Shoulders: Attempt to touch your ears with your shoulders.

Upper back: Push your shoulder blades together and stick out your chest.

Chest: Take a deep breath.

Stomach: Pull your stomach into your spine or push it out.

Lower Body

Buttocks: Tighten your buttocks and push into the chair.

Thighs: Straighten your legs and tighten your thigh muscles.

Calves: Point your toes toward your head.

Toes: Curl your toes—gently so they don't cramp.

Make sure to tense only the muscles in the area that you are studying while keeping other muscles relaxed. For example, to tense your biceps, you bend your arms at the elbow and make a "he-man" muscle. While doing this, let your hands hang limp. If you make a fist at the same time that you tense your biceps, you are tensing two muscle groups rather than one, which makes it harder to study the sensation of tension in the biceps.

Two Sensations

THE OBJECTIVE IS to discriminate between two feelings—tension and relaxation—so that you can recognize each. It is something like holding a heavy rock in one hand and a lighter rock in the other and "weighing" the two. Discriminating between a very heavy rock and a much lighter one is easy. By comparing the weight of one rock against the other you can learn to identify small differences in weight. You can train yourself to identify small changes in tension by studying the sensations in a tense muscle, then comparing that feeling to how the muscle feels when relaxed.

It takes about twenty-five minutes to go through your entire body slowly and systematically tensing and relaxing your muscles. You can develop an internal monitor by going through the exercise at least three times a week for two or three weeks. Study the more tension-prone areas, such as muscles in your face or shoulders, for five to seven minutes each day. In as short a time as two weeks, you will notice you are much more tuned into your activation level. The more you practice, the better your internal monitor will become.

The Relax Command

YOU CAN PROGRAM a "relax command" while you develop
your internal stress monitor. The actual command word
doesn't really matter. It can be any word, but "relax" is
good because it already has the association. When you're
tense, other people say, "Hey, Betty, come on and relax.
Just relax, girl." However, you might want to use a different word or words, such as "calm down," "quiet," "chill
out," or any word or phrase you prefer.

Program Your "Relax Command"

Step 1: Select a command word for programming

Step 2: Tense the practice muscle for 7 to 10 seconds.

Step 3: Think the command word just before quickly
releasing the tension from the muscle.

After selecting a word to use as a relax command, create
a strong and clear association between the command
word and the physiological sensations of relaxation.
The objective is to associate your word with the feeling
of *releasing* tension. As you systematically go through
the muscles in your body, tensing the muscles one at a
time, *think the command word, "Relax," just at the moment when you quickly release tension.* Each time you do
this, the association between the relax command and the
release of tension becomes stronger. Thinking the relax
command should come at the time of actually releasing
tension or just an instant before release.

Practice associating the command word with the
release of tension as follows. Tense the practice muscle

just enough to notice the tension. Hold the tension for about seven seconds while your study it, noticing how and where it feels. Then think your relax command just a moment before you quickly release the tension from the muscle. Allow the muscle to relax, and then do whatever it takes in your mind to push the muscle to relax just a little more. Study the sensations of relaxation as compared to that of tension. Practice one-by-one with each of the muscle groups.

The objective is to create a strong and clear association between the command word and your physical sensations of relaxation so that when you think the relax command your body relaxes.

Practice in a quiet spot for about two weeks, then slowly transfer the relaxation training into your daily routine. The key word here is *slowly*. If your first attempt to use the relax command is during a highly charged emotional encounter, you are likely to be disappointed in the result—because the situation will probably overwhelm the command and your confidence will drop.

In the course of the relaxation practice, you create new neural pathways for carrying messages to muscles, organs and their cells. When you stop to think about it, it is exciting—empowering—to realize that by systematically thinking your relax command and deliberately relaxing certain muscles, you can actually influence your cells.

Develop a Routine

IF YOU CAN, go through the tensing—relax command—relaxing slowly twice with each muscle during one practice session, which takes about twenty-five minutes. Strive to practice twice a day, once in the morning and once in the evening. It takes about two weeks of self-training to become relatively skilled at relaxing yourself when you want to do so.

Relax in Real Life

WHEN IN A TENSE SITUATION, focus attention on the tense muscles, take a deep breath and while holding it for three to six seconds, think your relax command, and then consciously relax the muscles. As with any skill you learn, go slowly and pat yourself on the back for small advances. Look for situations in which to practice and don't jump in over your head. Build your skill, solidly, step-by-step.

Slowly integrate the relaxation practice into your daily routine. Instead of a coffee break, which could increase your stimulation, you might close your office door, turn off the lights and spend five minutes practicing the relax command with one or two muscle groups. You might practice during times when you are stuck waiting for an elevator, or hanging on hold on the phone, or sitting in a waiting room. Next, use the relax command in mildly anxiety-provoking situations, such as before meeting with a supervisor.

Practicing relaxation is an ideal way to unwind for the evening. Instead of worrying, take a minute to relax before making a difficult phone call that you have been putting off. Remember, when you sense tension or catch yourself worrying, take a deep breath, focus on the tense muscle, think the relax command, and consciously release the tension.

Rock Yourself

REPETITIVE MOVEMENT, such as rocking, is soothing. When an infant cries, most people instinctively want to rock it. Even though you may think of rocking as being good only for little babies, it also has a powerful calming effect on adults. When you feel shaken up by worry, rocking yourself can soothe you, allowing the tension to drift away.

Engaging in a repetitive activity has a lulling, sometimes even a numbing effect. If you recall the movie *Rain Man*, the autistic man played by Dustin Hoffman often engaged in repetitive, rocking activities,   *Being rocked* such as stepping back and forth from one   *is soothing* foot to the other in a robot-like fashion as he said meaningless phrases over and over. While there is a lot of controversy surrounding autism, psychologists generally believe that the rocking and repetitively repeateing words and behavior serve to soothe the autistic person's extreme anxiety.

Repetitive Activity

REPETITIVE ACTIVITY is an effective relaxant for all people. Focusing your attention on a repetitive activity while passively disregarding intruding thoughts elicits the relaxation response.

Even though you are grown up and your mom is no longer around to rock you to sleep, you can always rock yourself to soothe and comfort yourself. Rocking can take many forms, but basically it is any repetitive back-and-forth motion. Rocking in a favorite rocking chair is a common self-rocking technique. Another enjoyable way to rock yourself is by swaying back and forth to music that has an even beat—which can be quick or slow,

because either is generally soothing. Or you can do a
simple exercise such as jumping jacks, stepping up and
down on a stair, or even jogging. If you are more seden-
tary, knitting or crocheting might be a good choice. These
"meditations-in-motion" soothe anxiety while lulling your
mind into letting go of stressful thoughts. Yes, the worrisome thinking will sneak back in, especially at first.
When it does, disregard it and bring your attention back
to the rocking.

Breathing

BREATHING IS SO NATURAL—and essential to life—that
we don't think of it as a tool we can use to operate our
bio-robot. But it is! Breathing seems to just happen, fast
when excited or frightened; slowly when sleeping. The
way you breathe has much to do with your level of tension or relaxation. In the next chapter, we will explore
the power of breathing, how to use it purposefully to relax, and how, in doing so skillfully, you can harness the
placebo effect.

10

Breathe

BREATHING IS THE MASTER KEY to self-healing, according to Andrew Weil, M.D., one of many proponents of using breath control to help the body heal itself. Breath is a method of controlling the body, regulating mental states, connecting the conscious and non-conscious parts of our brain, reducing anxiety, and even raising spiritual awareness.

Breath control works because in changing the way you breathe, you can rev the body up or calm it down. Stress is a primary or aggravating cause of many illnesses, physical and psychological. You can use breathing to counter the stress response. Stress produces a number of known bodily reactions, one of which is a specific type of fast, shallow breathing. In fact, if you breathe that way when you do *not* feel stressed, your body will begin to respond in stress-related ways, such as increased heart rate!

Try this now. First, notice how tense or relaxed you feel right now. Rate your feeling on a scale from 1 to 9, with 1 being very relaxed and calm, and with 9 being extremely tense and stressed out. Now breathe rapidly and shallowly, like a dog panting. Keep breathing rapidly for a minute or so. Then stop and rate how you feel after rapid breathing, on the same 1 to 9 scale.

What did you notice? How did you feel after rapid breathing as compared to how you felt before? It may be subtle, but if you are like most of us, you probably noticed that your tension level rose a little—in just one minute—just by breathing rapidly on purpose.

You deliberately breathed rapidly and in doing so you modified your tension level. You also modified your blood pressure and secretion of various hormones. You were "operating" your bio-robot. Rapid breathing revs up your robot; slow, deep breathing slows it down.

Two-Way Effects

THE EFFECTS OF VARIOUS CONDITIONS on our bodies work two ways. If we are amused and relaxed, we smile: amusement is the cause and smiling the effect. But researchers have also discovered that the reverse is true: if we smile even though we feel "down," our body responds as it would if we were amused and relaxed. This is a simple cure for mild cases of "the blues," but one that many of us do not think of—because it is hard to think of smiling when your feelings are in the dumps.

In the same vein, certain external circumstances affect our breathing in particular ways—causing us to take shallower and faster breaths when stressed, or deeper and slower ones when relaxed. Here too the reverse is true: breathing more deeply and slowly tells our body that we are relaxed, as well as directly relaxing muscles and slowing the flow of blood through intake of oxygen and breathing out of carbon dioxide. This results in the production of hormones that provide a more health-tropic environment for our cells, causing our cells to work in ways that keep us well.

Correcting Imbalance

THE POWER OF BREATH WORK comes from the way it coun-
teracts the imbalances of bodily processes that underlie
many disorders. Hypertension, for example, can result
from an overactive *sympathetic nervous system,* which
produces the fight-or-flight hormones cortisol, adrena-
line/epinephrine, and norepinephrine. These hormones
speed heart rate, raise blood pressure, slow digestion,
and divert blood circulation away from the surface of the
body to the interior. These are necessary conditions for
coping with an external threat.

In an emergency, it is important to maintain blood
flow to the brain. So digestion shuts down, because it is
not essential during an emergency. The same is true of
the immune function. When the alarm conditions persist
long-term—when we live in a constant state of emergency preparedness, goaded by the seemingly never-ending
irritations of modern life—we open ourselves to hypertension, digestive disturbances and diseases that take advantage of a weakened immune system.

You can reduce stress by purposefully changing the
way you breathe. Controlled breathing engages the *parasympathetic nervous system,* which releases hormones
that counteract the stress response and return the body
to a calmer, more-balanced state conducive to health. The
parasympathetic nervous system slows the heart rate,
lowers blood pressure, increases blood flow to the skin,
and increases movement of the digestive system.

Too Many Threats

IDEALLY THESE TWO OPERATING SYSTEMS work in balance—
the technical term is *homeostasis*—but for many of us,

over-activity of the sympathetic nervous system means our bodies are responding as if there is a constant external threat that never goes away. It is this constant sympathetic-nervous-system stimulation that can lead to anything from cold hands—because the skin is deprived of adequate blood flow—to disturbed heart function, such as irregular heartbeat. And these disturbances can lead to others—many reasons

Breathe more deeply, slowly, quietly and more regularly.

people go to the doctor have at their root an imbalance of these two systems. Breath work increases parasympathetic tone, helping bring the two systems back into balance. It gets to the root of the problem and goes directly to the imbalance in the nervous systems' functions, correcting it over time through gradual repetitive input.

Opening Channels

FOCUSING ATTENTION and working with breath opens the channels between the conscious mind and the non-conscious mind. You may have greater recall of dreams and easier access to altered states of consciousness. You can harmonize the influence that the mind has on the body. When you work with breath you are really working on both spheres—the body and the mind. Interestingly, in many languages, the words for breath and spirit are the same! The mental component of breath is a sense of rhythmic expansion and contraction, taking a small break from your flow of thoughts to put your mind briefly into a healing place.

You can develop breathing that is deeper, slower, quieter, and more regular. Start by paying attention to how you breathe now. Anytime you notice your breathing, try to make your breath deeper, slower, quieter. When you get angry or afraid, you breathe more shallowly; when you are upset, your breath may be noisy and irregular. When you are relaxed and harmonious, your breathing is deep, slow, quiet, and regular. Knowing this is important, because if you are upset, it is not so easy to tell yourself to "calm down"—but you *can* deliberately slow your breathing to be deeper, quieter and more regular, which *will* calm you down.

When you take a deep breath, your belly should move outward. *Try this now.* Put you hand on your abdomen—is it going out when you take a deep breath? Are you letting your belly expand? This is abdominal breathing. We often constrict the belly and don't let it expand freely when we breathe—but it is only when your abdomen expands that you are taking in a full volume of air.

When to Practice

PRACTICING BREATHING can be done at any time of day, but many people like to practice when they first get up in the morning. At the other end of the day, practicing breath work when going to bed helps to promote sleepiness and turn off sleep-disturbing thoughts. Many people practice breath work before meditating—although it is not necessary to practice meditation in order to get the benefits of breath work.

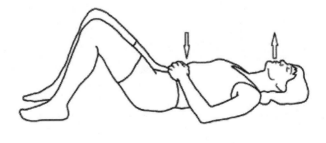

Set up a habit and practice every day. Change your breathing and you change rhythms in your nervous system, which takes time. Constancy and regularity of practice helps the body learn the changes. The power of breath work is like the power of water cutting a canyon—constant gentle force over time produces big results. So find times in the day that suit you and feel natural, and then make a resolution to practice your breath work at those times.

Breathing practice is easy and takes only a few minutes a day. You will enjoy it. You will experience results over the space of a few weeks: real changes in your energy level, in your sleep patterns, in your digestion and circulation, in stress levels.

How to Start

To BEGIN WITH, just sit. Use a comfortable chair to keep your back straight—wear loose clothing. Sit in a quiet place. Close your eyes or keep them open or half-closed—whatever makes you comfortable.

Follow Your Breath

SIMPLY PAY ATTENTION to your breathing—do not try to change it in any way. Don't speed it up or slow it down—just follow it. Notice the cycles of inhalation and exhalation. Notice how your breath flows. Your attention may wander. This is normal; we all get distracted. Just bring your attention back to your breathing. When it wanders again, gently bring your attention back to your breath again and again. Focus on your breath—in and out, inhalation and exhalation. Don't try to influence it; just keep your attention on your breathing.

When observing your breath, where do you notice it? In your nostrils? In your throat? In your chest as it expands? In your abdomen expanding? There is no one right way to observe. The key is to pay attention, to familiarize yourself with the way you breathe.

Reverse the Breath Cycle

IN THIS EXERCISE, start by doing your usual breathing in and out, in and out, in and out. Then stop. Now begin each breath with the exhalation, so you breathe out and then in. Out and in. Out and in. Do this for a few minutes. Don't try to influence your breath—don't try to speed it up or slow it down. Just breathe out and then in, out and in for a minute or two. Again, just follow your breath that begins with an out-breath and ends with an in-breath. In doing this exercise, you take greater control of your breathing by increasing the amount of air that you move out.

Squeeze More Air Out

THE SECRET OF BREATH CONTROL is increasing the exhalation step. When you squeeze more air *out* you automatically take more air *in*. Use the muscles between the ribs to squeeze air out. Feel the muscular effort as you squeeze. Take a deep breath in through your nose, then let it out through your mouth. When you get to the end, squeeze a little more air out. Then squeeze a little more out. Notice the effort it takes? Feel it in your ribs?

Whenever you notice your breathing, squeeze a little more air out on the exhalation. Most people put effort into the inhalation and very little effort into exhaling. You can deepen and lengthen exhalation with this exercise— by moving more air in and out of your lungs.

Stimulating Breath

THIS EXERCISE HELPS RAISE ENERGY in the nervous system
and increases awareness. It may increase your body
temperature as well. The process is to breathe in rapidly through your nose, with your mouth lightly closed.
Inhalation and exhalation will both be short and fast.
This produces rapid movement of the diaphragm, which
simulates the movement of a bellows and makes a noisy
breath sound.

Try it the first time for only about fifteen seconds—it
takes practice! Then breathe normally again. You can increase the time by a few seconds in each practice, slowly,
until you can do bellows breathing for about a minute.
Notice how you feel when you finish the exercise. This is
a good technique for waking yourself up if you feel sleepy
or drowsy from mental fatigue—or when driving.

After breath work, it is a good idea to sit quietly, maybe listen to music—just enjoy being in a peaceful, meditative state, even if you do not practice formal meditation. Controlled breathing *is* a gateway to meditation and
can help you enter and remain in a meditative state. You
feel peaceful as it engages your parasympathetic nervous
system, which operates at the non-conscious level to tell
your body to produce more hormones that allow your
cells to behave in a health-tropic manner.

The Four Qualities

WHENEVER YOU NOTICE YOUR BREATHING, take a moment
to practice making your breathing deeper, slower, quieter, and more even. These are the four qualities you are
striving to develop with breath work. First observe your
breath for a minute. Then consciously make your breath

deeper, slower, quieter and more regular. When you get upset or knocked off-balance, take as many breaths as you can while making them deeper, slower, quieter and more regular. In doing this, you will make your body function better and will quiet your mind, harmonizing your nervous system right down to your cells. Remember: deeper, slower, quieter, more regular.

The Universe Breathes

IMAGINE THAT YOU ARE NOT BREATHING but that the Universe is breathing *through* you. Feel the breath coming into your body and into every cell. Imagine your breath coming into your lungs and going out to every cell in your body, nourishing those cells and energizing them. It helps to put your tongue on the small ridge behind your teeth on the roof of your mouth. Exhale from your mouth around your tongue to make a *whoosh* sound.

Exhale though your mouth completely. Hear the whoosh. Then inhale quietly though your nose, to a count of four. Hold your breath, to a count of seven. Then exhale from your mouth to a count of eight. Repeat this four times—each repeat is one cycle. In the beginning, practice with four cycles of this breathing exercise.

According to Dr. Weil, keeping the ratio is important: inhalation count 4, hold count 7, and exhale count 8. The maximum time is not important, but the ratio of the breathing matters—it is the ratio that is helping you control your breathing. As you practice, using this ratio, you will get better and better at this form of breathing—more and more able to slow your body down on the inside.

When you are done with the 4-7-8 cycle, breath normally, without trying to influence your breath. Just notice how you feel. If you are like most people, you will feel deeply relaxed. Some people feel a little light-headed; this will disappear with more practice. As you practice, the process becomes easier and easier. Practice four breath cycles twice a day. After a month, if you are comfortable, increase to eight breath cycles per practice—but never more than eight each practice. In your everyday life, when you find yourself getting upset about something, do a few breath cycles before you react. Practicing breath control can quell anxiety as well as help control cravings, such as the desire to smoke when you are quitting.

When first beginning breath work, you may find it helpful to follow a guide. Weil's audio program, *Breathing: The Master Key to Self-Healing*, is one such. Or enter the terms "breath work" or "breathing exercises" into a search engine—there are many programs and approaches available. Experiment until you find one that you feel good about practicing and enjoy.

11

Get Good Sleep

Y OU KNOW YOU NEED SLEEP, yet you scrimp on sleeping. It's become a lifestyle. Maybe you did "all-nighters" preparing for exams in college. On road trips, you may push late into the night, keeping awake with coffee and energy drinks. If you're a parent, you probably sacrifice sleep when family demands mount. In the process, you cheat yourself of the benefit of your body's reparative properties during sleep. You cheat your cells out of prime healing conditions.

Sleep deprivation has become the new normal. We live in a 24/7 society. But is that good? One in three American adults is sleep-deprived according to the Centers for Disease Control and Prevention (CDC). About 20% of Americans report that they get less than 6 hours of sleep a night on average. The National Sleep Foundation estimates that 50 to 70 million U.S. adults have sleep or wakefulness disorders. Sleep deficit is linked to poor work performance, driving accidents, relationship problems, and mood difficulties, such as anger and depression. Obesity has also been linked to chronic sleep loss.

Sleep deprivation is the new normal

Sleep-deprived drivers are as dangerous as drunk drivers. The Department of Transportation estimates that more than 100,000 crashes with 1,550 fatalities and

40,000 nonfatal injuries annually in the United States are due to driving while drowsy. Sleep deprivation reduces the ability to make split-second decisions. Sleep-deprived people have problems with categorization, which involves analyzing incoming information in order to makes decisions and act accordingly. Ability to categorize declines steeply when we are sleep deprived, meaning we make poor decisions and react too slowly—an obvious danger when driving.

Lack of sleep affects health in numerous ways, but sleep-deprived people often don't realize their vulnerability. Getting insufficient sleep sets you up for disease. You give your body too little time to regenerate. Soon there are breakdowns.

Increased Blood Pressure

PEOPLE WITH HIGH BLOOD PRESSURE are more prone to cardiovascular disease if they don't get enough sleep. Lack of enough sleep may cause hypertension in adults, according to a study in journal *Archives of Internal Medicine*. Research has shown stress hormones tend to be elevated in people who are sleep deprived.

Weight Gain

CHRONIC LOSS of three hours of sleep per night goes along with increased consumption of calories, which go right to the waistline. Irregular sleep patterns and sleeping during daylight are correlated with a higher risk of colon and breast cancer, according to a Harvard Medical School study. Researchers point to insufficient melatonin, a hormone produced during sleep in dark environments, that combats the growth of tumor cells.

Depression

ONGOING LACK OF SLEEP heightens risk of depression. Disrupted sleep can lead to anxiety and intrusive thoughts, sometimes called "the monkey mind." People sleeping less than seven hours a night are twice as likely to have a major depressive episode.

Dullness

WHEN YOUR SLEEP is frequently interrupted, your brain spends less time in the much-needed REM (Rapid Eye Movement) state, which is when most dreaming occurs. As a result, you feel sluggish and have trouble performing tasks and remembering things.

Why don't we get enough sleep? The biggest sleep stopper is stress—and an inability to turn off nighttime worrying. Many people are kept awake by a physical problem, such as chronic pain or allergies. Some struggle with factors in their sleep environment—a snoring spouse, a young child crying. It is important to find ways to overcome these obstacles to restful sleep, because increased nightly sleep improves memory, increases the ability to concentrate, strengthens the immune system, and decreases the risk of being injured in accidents.

Get Better Sleep

THERE ARE THINGS YOU CAN DO to increase the chance of getting better sleep.

Be Tired at Bedtime

STAY OUT OF BED until you are tired. Lying in bed waiting to fall asleep can lead to sleep anxiety, making it harder to doze off. Engaging in calm and quiet activity, such as reading or listening to relaxing music before bedtime, promotes sleep. Avoid television and bright lights. If you can't fall asleep, get out of bed and engage in a boring activity, such as polishing silver or sorting papers, until you're drowsy.

Bed Limits

USE YOUR BED only for sex and sleep. Train your mind and body to associate the bed with rest and relaxation, not with watching TV, surfing the Internet, eating a snack, or working. Treat your bed like a bed, not a desk.

Follow a Nightly Ritual

GO TO BED around the same time every night. Create a relaxing bedtime routine to help prepare your mind and body for sleep. A hot bath or shower, soft music, dim lights, and pleasant fragrances help you relax for sleep. When you follow a nightly routine, the ritual becomes a cue telling your body it's time to sleep.

Exercise Lightly

AN EASY EXERCISE SESSION after work, ideally between 5 and 7 p.m., will leave you feeling calm, prepping you for dreamland. Regular exercise is a general sleep promoter. Engage in aerobic exercise on most days of the week, at whatever time of day is convenient for you. You do not have to work out right before bedtime to tire your body—in fact, some people find that exercising too close to bedtime makes it harder to drift off because they are still revved up.

Eat Early

AVOID EATING during the three hours before bed, and limit alcohol to just one glass (for women) or two (for men) with dinner. Too much alcohol may make you sleepy at first, but it will interfere with your sleep cycle in the night.

Deal with Snoring

SNORING CAN BE A SYMPTOM of sleep apnea, which is a decrease of airflow during sleep. It can be difficult to sleep soundly with a snorer causing you to wake up frequently throughout the night. Encourage your snoring sleep partner to talk to a physician about taking a sleep test to diagnose the condition. Bringing sleep apnea under control will mean more-restful nights.

Avoid Electronic Gadgets

LIGHT FROM ELECTRONIC DEVICES such as computers, cell phones and televisions stimulates the brain, keeping you awake. Lights suppress melatonin, so sleep in a dark room or use a sleep mask. If your clock shows blue numbers, that light could block melatonin production and keep you awake. Pick a clock that emits amber light, or adopt your grandmother's wind-up ticker.

Get Out of Bed

IF YOU CAN'T FALL ASLEEP within 20 minutes or so, get out of bed, go into another room, and read or listen to music in low light. But no TV, which tends to keep you awake. When you are feeling sleepy, go back to bed. This not only keeps you from getting frustrated as you toss and turn but also helps your body associate the bed with sleep, not wakefulness.

Keep Your Bedroom Cool

KEEP THE TEMPERATURE of your bedroom between 65 and
72 degrees Fahrenheit to help cool your body's core temperature to a comfortable sleeping level.

Try a Soothing Scent

A WHIFF OF LAVENDER before bed helps some people sleep
more deeply. Don't rely on synthetic scents—they create
indoor air pollution and may contain harmful chemicals.
Instead, fill a spray bottle with water and add two or
three drops of organic lavender essential oil, and spritz
the bedroom before you hit the sack.

Take Smart Naps

RESEARCHERS HAVE FOUND that people who take an after-
noon nap are able to learn more afterwards. Taking a
short nap refreshes your brain and increases your ability
to learn new information. According to research from the
University of California at Berkeley, "the capacity of the
brain to learn facts is improved by sleep," explains lead
researcher Matt Walker, Ph.D. Walker says that naps of
five to 10 minutes help refresh alertness. "Sleep both
before and after learning has been shown to improve
memory—before, to get your brain ready for learning, and
after, to solidify what you have just learned.

Thus, proper sleeping habits are critical." Experiment
to find what nap length works best for you. People generally perform more sharply and function better right after a
10-minute nap. Do not nap for too long—you will go into
REM sleep and may find it hard to wake up and quickly
resume normal activities.

Talk to your doctor

IF YOUR DOCTOR doesn't bring it up, start the conversation yourself. Your doctor should assess your sleep behaviors to determine if treatment is needed and how sleep is affecting any other medical issues.

Sleep is a part of overall health, and sleep disturbances can be very damaging. Sleep disorders are severely under-diagnosed and under-treated.

Sleep is restorative, allowing your health-tropic cells to regain energy lost during the day and letting your brain, at a non-conscious level, manage those cells to maximize health and fight off any potential illnesses. Sleep deprivation makes it easier for ever-present environmental threats, such as viruses, to gain a foothold in your body and move it away from wellness.

There is a reason that we are biologically programmed to spend about one-third of our lives asleep: sleep is an absolute necessity for maintenance of health and restoration of wellness. Yet sleep is often the first thing we sacrifice in the name of getting more work done, spending more time at entertainment events, or pushing ourselves in other ways.

To engage the placebo effect and keep ourselves well, we need an attitude adjustment that restores sleep to the level of importance that our biology gives it. Think seriously about ways you have cut into your sleep time and find methods of restoring the amount of sleep your body needs—and talk to your doctor if sleep problems persist.

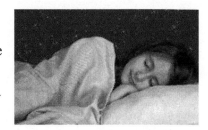

12

Healing Power of Dreams

DREAMS HAVE FASCINATED PEOPLE from the beginning of recorded history. The ancients looked to dreams for healing power. Pilgrims traveled to dream temples hoping to receive a dream in which a healing god would appear in the dream to cure them or give them advice about a problem.

It seems pretty clear that through dreams we somehow communicate with a non-conscious part of our minds. Sigmund Freud's first breakthrough in creating psychotherapy was *The Interpretation of Dreams*, in which he argued that dreams are an expression of disguised wish fulfillment. Fascination with dreams and their interpretation continues today.

Candace Pert, Ph.D., author of *Molecules of Emotion*, is a biophysics and physiology researcher who believes, "Dreams are direct messages from your body-mind, giving you valuable information about what's going on physiologically as well as emotionally. Strong emotions that are not processed thoroughly are stored at the cellular level. At night some of the stored information is released and allowed to bubble up into consciousness as a dream. Capturing the dream and re-experiencing the emotions can be very healing, as you either integrate the information for growth or decide to take actions toward forgiveness and letting go."

Dreams and Wellness

HARNESSING YOUR DREAMS can be an important part of
engaging the placebo effect, allowing your health-tropic
cells to move in the direction of wellness in which they
naturally want to go. But many of us find the notion of
"using" dreams counter-intuitive, believing that dreams
"just happen" and are not strongly integrated with brain
function. This is a fundamental misunderstanding of
dreaming.

While it is true that researchers have shown that certain parts of the brain go "offline" during dreaming, it is
also true that other parts of the brain go on "high speed
access." PET (positive emission tomography) studies
show that the limbic and paralimbic systems of the brain
are activated during REM sleep (Rapid Eye Movement,
when most dreams occur). Activated areas include the
amygdala, hippocampus, parahippocampal cortex, ante-
rior cingulate, and medial prefrontal cortex.

Robert Hoss, author of *Dream Language*, says that
the limbic system mediates emotional experience, emotional behavior and conversion of emotions into physiology. The right hypothalamus, which integrates senso-
ry-perceptual, emotional and cognitive functions of the
mind with the biology of the body, is also active. At the
same time, there is a loss of
functional connection be-
tween the frontal cortex and
posterior perceptual areas,
which is believed to result
in a lack of reality testing—
hence different types of brain
communications.

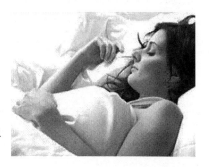

What Dreaming Does

EMOTIONAL PROCESSING seems to be a function of dreaming. During dreaming the activated areas of the brain communicate in different ways than during waking consciousness, allowing emotions to be processed differently. The limbic system speaks in the language of symbolic imagery. Working with dream imagery in the waking state can help change perceptions and resolve conflicts, which are critical keys for healing because the mind communicates with the body through imagery.

It is significant that the amygdala and hypothalamus, which are both highly active during dreaming, have forty times as many opiate and neuropeptide receptors as other parts of the brain. Mark Weisberg, Ph.D., in *The Power of Mind-Body Medicine*, says that dreams positively impact these receptors, and they in turn can have a positive impact on the immune system.

The amygdala is thought to assign emotional significance to the data it receives. Take, for instance, our reaction to scary movies—or scary dreams. The event may not really be threatening, but the amygdala perceives the danger as real and triggers chemical changes in the body as though it were real; without this, horror films would not scare us at all, nor would nightmares. This part of the brain doesn't know a real event from a perceived event—and this is how perception can change biology, because the non-conscious accepts all that it received as "real."

Getting Past Filters

DREAMS ARE A WAY of getting past our conscious filters to our underlying biology—and we can train ourselves to use dreams to help us get well and stay well. For example:

- Dreams show us emotions we may have ignored in waking life.

- Dreams show us how we create stresses in our lives.

- Dreams put us in touch with our personal conflicts.

- Dreams show us potential new responses.

Through dreams, you can cut through conscious resistance; and because of the parts of the brain that are inactive during dreaming, you can cut through waking logic, to let limbic logic take over.

Nightmares are useful, too. They are dreams that give us a "heads up" and show us where we are out of balance and in need of repair. Scary dreams show us something we have ignored, repressed or denied. The best response to a nightmare is to muse upon it to determine its message. Helping nightmare imagery evolve into more positive, healing imagery is a process by which you can actively participate in your own healing. Remember that we communicate non-consciously with our cells through images, not words.

Decode Dream Images

BY DECODING DREAM IMAGES that indicate the conditions of body parts and systems, you can get into closer touch with your body, down to the cells. A vital step is to create a Dream Journal for recording dreams and then to "re-dream" unhealthy images to change them into healthy ones. By writing about your nightmares—even sometimes adding pictures—you can release the trauma that your nightmares express. Many healers believe that visualizing your dream images of healing speeds your recovery, and much research supports this. Dreaming is a way to reach around the conscious brain to your body and cells to encourage them to work in harmony to heal.

Patricia Garfield, Ph.D., author of *The Healing Power of Dreams*, says that our dreams can help to keep us healthy. Dreams warn us when we are at risk. They can help to diagnose physical problems, provide support during physical crises, and forecast recuperation by suggesting treatments. Dreams have the power to help heal the body and signal our return to wellness. Of course dream-related treatment should never be a substitute for the advice of your doctor and appropriate medical treatment. But dreams can provide a resource that you can call upon when you are ill or have had an accident because, after all, your body is alive and intelligent—in the sense that your mind knows what is going on inside your body. You can learn how to tap into this knowledge, and dreaming is one way of doing so.

Dreams speak to us when we learn to listen to them. Most of us spend about 25% of our time when we are asleep, or about 90 minutes to two hours a night, in REM sleep. The final REM period in the night usually lasts about 30-45 minutes, and it is from this dream period that most of us remember dreams. (Dreams can also occur in non-REM periods.)

The Dream Plan

HERE'S WHAT TO DO. Don't judge the images and events in your dreams—just accept whatever comes. Plan for recalling your dreams before going to bed. Put a pad and pen, or a digital recorder, on the nightstand. Suggest to yourself as you are drifting off to sleep, "Tonight I will remember a dream." You might even picture yourself recording your dream.

Allow yourself to awaken spontaneously rather than with an alarm, which is disruptive. When you awaken, just lie still and allow the dream images to float through your mind. Use these to pull in more images from the dream. Record these images on your pad or on the recorder while keeping your eyes closed and all lights off, if possible. When writing, use your finger to guide the pen to prevent writing over the same place. Don't try to analyze or understand the dream while you are recording it. Just remember it and write it down.

Usually you should record things in the order you recall them, except when they have to do with phrases and words, like poems or names. Write these down right away because dream words are easily lost. Keep your eyes closed as long as you can because opening them can disrupt your recall.

If a dream comes to your memory during the day, record it as soon as you can. Later in the day, transcribe the initial record into a more permanent and organized record in a notebook or on your computer. Some people like using index cards.

Before going to sleep, put a date in your permanent record and jot down what you did and how you felt during that day. These notes become "facts" to go along with the dream. Include the salient events and feelings you experienced that day. When recording your dream into the permanent record, use the present tense—this will help you get back into the feeling of the dream. Give each dream a title based upon some feature in it. You

may want to make sketches or diagrams to illustrate aspects of the dream. Don't rush this. Just enjoy recalling
the dream and making notes in the permanent record.

Garfield says that dreams are problem-solving devices. As you grow in understanding your dreams, you will
get better at using these inner tools for guidance with
problems. In your recording of the dreams, make sure
you always include the feelings and emotions that you
had during the dream. These are important. As you gather descriptions and read them over, notice connection
between your dream feelings and your waking feelings.
Ideas in your waking life may come to you as you are
writing down description of images and elements in your
dream journal. Make sure to write these down as well, to
help connect the dream world with your waking world.

How to Analyze

THE WAY TO ANALYZE DREAMS is through the associations
that the dream images bring to mind. Take the main
action of the dream. What is the oddest thing in the
dream? If there was a person, who was it? What was special about him or her? If that image could speak, what
would it say? What were the colors and other elements in
the dream? What do these bring to mind?

The approach is to notice what you *associate* with the
image—what it brings to mind. Amplify the images in
the dream, especially anything that brought up a strong
emotion. Make connections: first make an association
with what comes to mind with key images, then substitute these associations for the images and actions in the
dream. A message will begin to emerge, almost as if you
were making a translation from a foreign language. It's
exciting, really.

Images in our dreams are metaphors. With a metaphor, one thing is likened to another, different thing—there is an implied comparison. We speak in metaphors all the time, not just in writing and dreams, but also in our everyday talking with others. We use images in everything we say. What is special about dream images is that they are metaphors for our emotions—a kind of picture language of how we feel. Dreams of falling, for example, may symbolize feeling disappointed or failing in a project.

The dreaming mind may see lack of emotional support as failure. In musing on this you may say, "He let me down." Another example: an animal with sharp teeth might symbolize anger. You may have pent-up anger or be worried about someone who may be angry with you. You might dream of biting and a scary animal because you think of being wounded with words. Dreaming of drowning or being buried in snow can represent feeling overwhelmed—just as, in everyday discourse, you may sometimes talk about "drowning in work" or being "snowed under."

Body Metaphors

THE TWO MOST COMMON METAPHORS for bodies are houses and vehicles. With a few moments' thought it is easy to see how a house is much like a body: both contain all kinds of pipes and tubes. The comparison—the metaphor—is easy to understand. A staircase in a dream might represent the spine. Windows might represent eyes. The back door might be an anus. Pipes might be blood vessels. Electrical wires could be nerves. Often, although of course not always, when there is a cottage or a castle or a house in a dream, it symbolizes one's own body. A barn with animals might symbolize a woman being pregnant, with unborn children in the womb.

If, when you dream about a house, there is an emphasis on the structure of the house, this may be referring to your body as a metaphor. So pay attention. What is the house like? Is it cared for and attractive—or in need of repair? Is there something broken and disconnected? Is the house attractive and harmonious or ugly? Is the foundation strong or crumbling? Are there hidden rooms? Often these metaphors can reveal something about the connections in your body. And those connections are not limited to the physical: the dream can be speaking about the psychological as well.

Vehicle Images

OTHER COMMON DREAM IMAGES for the body are vehicles—trucks, cars, trains, boats. These tend to symbolize your body in action. The car is the most common vehicle in dreams today. As with houses, the parallel between bodies and vehicles is easy to see. They both consume fuel: we eat and cars use gas. Both excrete wastes, and both have insides and outsides. Dreams about vehicles focus more on the body's functioning than on the body's structure. A steering wheel, for instance, might refer to direction—if you dream that you cannot steer, that may mean you feel your life is out of control. Brakes may represent control of activity.

Headlights can symbolize eyes. Fuel can be energy. Tires and wheels can be legs. When you dream of a vehicle, pay close attention to its details. What kind of vehicle? A sports car? Sedan? Old? New? What is its condition? Are you at the steering wheel? If not, who is? Is it moving fast or slowly? Do the brakes work? How does it drive on the road? Perhaps it has been in an accident. Are the tires okay? Are there any malfunctioning parts?

What is the outside like? Is it polished? Is there enough gas in the tank? Where is the car going—to somewhere good, somewhere bad, somewhere unknown? Think of all these elements as metaphors for how your body is functioning.

Organs

EACH ORGAN IN THE BODY has a voice in dreams. You may dream of eating a delicious meal and awaken to find yourself very hungry. Men commonly awaken from a passion dream with an erection. Most people have had dreams of wanting to urinate and then wake to find they need to go to the bathroom. These normal bodily functions translate into dreams—and in the same way, abnormal processes or illnesses can be revealed to you.

Certain dysfunctions in our organs and bodies can be intertwined in a dream story. For example, people who develop a headache during sleep may dream of images revolving around damage or injury to the head—such as being hit on the head with various things, being attacked by animals that do things to one's head, wearing constricting head gear, finding one's head on fire, and so forth.

Incubate Healing Dreams

YOU CAN INCUBATE A DREAM for healing. In psychological terms, incubation is defined as a process of unconscious recombination of thought elements that were stimulated through conscious work at one point in time, resulting in novel ideas at some later point in time. In dreaming, incubation is stimulated with a question, such as "how can I heal myself?" or "how can I get well?" The question or request should be concise and phrased in words meaningful to you.

After deciding upon your question or request, pick a day and a time when you feel relaxed and can concentrate on the question. Look at pictures and books, and engage in activities relevant to your question. Repeat your incubation request several times and think about it during the day. Remind yourself of your goal for the coming night's dream. Write your incubation request in your dream journal, with notes on how you feel and your activities during the day.

At bedtime, as you begin drifting off to sleep, chant your request softly in your mind. As you fall asleep, picture yourself in a state in which your request is being fulfilled. Leave yourself open to whatever the dream may provide. Then in the morning, or even in the night if you wake up, make sure to have easy access to a pad and pen or a recorder next to your bed. Record your dream so that you can explore it later as an answer to your question.

Because dreams use metaphors, many initially seem to have no connection at all to the incubation question or request. Yet as you study and work through the images in the dream, consider the associations the dream calls up, and muse upon the images to see feelings and inspirations they bring into your conscious mind—thinking of the dream as an overall message or possible answer— you will often find a profound connection. And if you can find no connection at all, do not worry! Just repeat the attempt. Sometimes it may take three or four nights, or even more, to get a clear dream answer. In fact, sometimes a vivid dream answer will come after you stop trying so hard.

Dream solutions and advice may come in many ways—maybe involving a food to eat or an activity to engage in. And the solutions can be applied to minor everyday issues or to major ones involving significant health threats. O. Carl Simonton, M.D., an internationally known oncologist, pioneered research in psychosocial oncology, using a model of emotional support for the treatment of cancer patients—an approach that introduced the concept that one's state of mind could influence the ability to survive cancer. This involved, among other things, visualizing, consciously and through dreams, improvements in health—a technique that we all can use whenever we are feeling subpar or simply looking for better balance in our lives to give our cells a chance to assert their natural health-tropic inclination. The point is that this is the power of dreams—they are a way to reach down to the cells in your body to communicate your healing message for the body to implement.

13

Meditate

MEDITATING RESTS THE MIND, allowing it to rejuvenate. In meditation, you watch your thoughts
from a detached perspective and in *the process train
your attention*. This is very powerful. You learn to direct
your thoughts and mood—an ability that has profound
self-healing implications for physical and mental health.

Meditation calms the mind, promoting inner peace
and, with practice, reaching a higher spiritual dimen-
sion, referred to simply as *being*. People have different
reasons for wanting to meditate, from quelling internal
chatter, getting to know oneself better, finding calm and
a sense of grounding, to enforced restful contemplation.

Studying the brainwaves of meditating monks, Dr.
Richard Davidson, director of the Laboratory for Affective
Neuroscience at the University of Wisconsin, found that
brain circuitry is different in long-time meditators from
that in non-meditators. Certain regions of the brain—the
amygdala and the right prefrontal cortex—are activated
when we are upset: anxious, depressed, angry. When
we are in a positive mood, the *left* prefrontal cortex—a
region associated with happiness
and positivity—becomes more active. Meditating monks had especially high activity in this area.

*Meditation calms
the mind, promoting
inner peace.*

The brain can rewire itself and alter its set points through the self-healing power of thought. Quantum biologist Bruce Lipton says deep relaxation changes our bodies on a genetic level. The relaxation response can be as powerful as pharmaceutical drugs but without the side effects. Herbert Benson, M.D., of Harvard Medical School, found that a range of disease-fighting genes were active in those practicing meditation.

When we are stressed, our heart rate rises and our blood pressure shoots up. Muscles contract and tighten. Immunity, digestion and other non-essential functions become secondary. By contrast, relaxation is a state of rest, enjoyment and physical renewal. Feeling safe, muscles relax and food is digested. Heart rate slows and blood circulation flows, feeding tissues and cells with nutrients and oxygen.

There are many methods of meditating. Guided meditation is a popular approach. You might work with a teacher or guide, or a pre-made recording, taking yourself on a journey to a place you find calming or relaxing. Transcendental meditation employs a mantra, which is a word or phrase that you repeat over and over to yourself silently to prevent distracting thoughts from entering. In mindful meditation, you focus acutely on your surroundings—inner and outer—while breathing deeply and watching your feelings without judgment. Mediation methods may be different, but they all lead to deep relaxation.

How to Meditate

PICK A PLACE where you will not be interrupted. Being there should feel calm and peaceful, which will enable you to focus on your meditation without being interrupted by outside stimuli. The space does not need to be very large so long as it is somewhere private. Make sure to turn off TV sets, cell phones and any noisy appliances. You may want to try out various places before settling on one.

Complete silence is not necessary. Background sounds, such as an occasional dog bark, lawn mower, church bell, or passing car, won't prevent effective meditation and are actually helpful, because being aware of noises but not letting them intrude is important in learning to meditate.

Playing music that is calming, repetitive and gentle is a popular approach and can be helpful, especially for those new to meditation. Meditating near running water or a water fountain is also a favorite experience, because the sound of running water can be extremely calming.

Experiment with meditating outside. Pick a peaceful place, such as under a tree, in a meadow with lush grass, or atop a stone outcropping. Being in nature helps, especially for spiritual enhancement.

Wear Comfortable Clothes

SHOES PINCHING YOUR TOES or a belt digging into your back will draw your attention to the discomfort, which will fight your efforts to calm your mind. Wear loose clothing during meditation practice, and remove your shoes or wear slippers. Wear a sweater or jacket when it is somewhat cool so that the sensation of being cold doesn't intrude, tempting you to cut your practice short. If at work, open the collar of your shirt or blouse and remove your belt.

Sit in a Comfortable Position

TRADITIONALLY, meditation is practiced by sitting on a cushion on the ground or in a yoga position called "lotus," which, however, takes very flexible legs and hips for comfort. If this is not possible or comfortable for you, experiment with sitting positions, on a cushion, chair, or meditation bench.

Your spine should be centered over the two bony bits in your buttocks—the spots that bear your weight—so your pelvis needs to be tilted forward. One way to tilt your pelvis into the right position is to sit on the forward edge of a thick cushion or chair, with a 3 or 4 inch thick board or stack of books under the back of the cushion or rear legs of the chair.

Then, starting from your buttocks, stack up the vertebrae in your spine, so that they are balanced one on top of another to support the weight of your torso, neck, and head. With practice you'll find the position that allows you to relax your torso, needing a slight effort to maintain your balance. Whenever you feel tension anywhere, relax the area. The most important thing is that you are comfortable, relaxed, and your torso is balanced so that your spine supports all of your weight from the waist up.

Experiment with sitting positions, on a cushion, chair, or meditation bench.

Rest your hands on your knees, leave them hanging down by your side, or use the traditional hand placement of hands in your lap, palms facing upward, with your right hand on top of your left.

Develop a Routine

MEDITATE AT THE SAME TIME every day so that it becomes part of your everyday routine. This way you will do it naturally, rather than constantly feeling that you must find time, which tends to generate resistance and procrastination. The best meditators are steady in their practice, doing it every day without exception.

Seasoned meditators agree early in the morning, shortly after getting up, is a good time to meditate. Your mind is already fresh from sleep, before you become consumed with the stresses of the day. Meditate before breakfast if in the morning, because fullness and the digestive process can be distracting.

Close Eyes at First

MEDITATION CAN BE PERFORMED with the eyes open or closed. Meditating with your eyes closed is best in the beginning to block out visual stimulation that will distract your efforts to calm your mind. After you've developed a little skill, you might try meditating with your eyes open, which can be helpful when falling asleep. Use a "soft" gaze—not focusing on anything in particular—when meditating with open eyes. Looking at a gazing ball, which is a mirrored globe, or at a candle flame can be helpful.

Breating Meditation

BREATHING MEDITATION is a basic meditation and a great place to start your practice. Focus your mind on a spot just above your navel and become aware of the rising and falling of that spot, that place on your abdomen, as you breathe in and out. Breathe normally and don't make any effort to

Breathe more deeply, slowly, quietly and more regularly.

change your breathing patterns. Just watch your breathing without analyzing it or trying to change it. Just be aware of your breathing.

Try this now. Loosen any binding clothing. Sit towards the front of your chair so your back is straight. Close your eyes and check in on yourself. Notice your level of tension and rate it on a scale of 1 to 9, with 1 being completely relaxed and 9 being extremely tense. Now imagine a spot or picture a coin just above your navel and focus your attention on it. Notice how it rises and falls with your breathing. Just keep watching the spot or coin rise and fall with your breathing. It is natural and to be expected that your mind will wander. When it does, don't scold yourself. Instead, just bring your attention back to the spot or coin rising and falling with your breath. Continue following your breath for one to two minutes, or longer.

When finishing your breathing meditation, just sit and notice how you feel. Again, rate your level of tension on a scale of 1 to 9, with 1 being completely relaxed and 9 being extremely tense. How do your ratings compare? How tense or relaxed do you feel now, after meditating on your breath for only one to two minutes, compared to how you felt before the meditation? Probably you notice a difference. If you're like most of us, you feel noticeably more relaxed now than before experimenting with the breathing meditation.

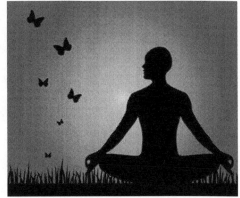

© passiflora70 - Fotolia.com

Mental pictures, such as imagining a coin above your navel, are a form of thinking and can be helpful in focusing attention. Another helpful image might be to imagine a buoy floating in the ocean, bobbing up and down with the swell and lull of your breathing.

Repeat a Mantra

MANTRA MEDITATION involves saying a mantra—a sound, word or phrase—over and over repetitively, until you silence you mind and enter a deep meditative state. The word *mantra* means "instrument of the mind" in Sanskrit. The mantra is an instrument that helps you to drive your thoughts away and enter a relaxed state of consciousness.

The mantra can be anything. *Om*, pronounced "ooooo-ummmm" while breathing out slowly, is widely used. Your mantra can be a phrase: "God is great; God is good," for example. You might use a favorite affirmation, such as "Every day I am getting better and better." It can be a sound without meaning, like "eeeing." The mantra meditation is simply silently repeating your mantra over and over to yourself.

Try mantra meditation now. Use the mantra "I am healing" for this trial. Make yourself comfortable, by loosening your clothing if needed. Sit up straight and close your eyes. As before, notice and rate *Try the mantra* your tension level on the 1 to 9 scale. *"I am healing."* Begin by breathing in slowly and deeply. Hold your breath for a second and begin saying your mantra to yourself, matching it to your breath as you breathe out slowly. "I am healing. Iyeeeeeee aaammm heeeaalinnnnng." Then breathe in the breath of life deeply, pause briefly, and exhale slowly while telling yourself over and over, "I am healing."

Expect your mind to wan-
der. This is natural. Without any
judgment, just bring your mind
back to your mantra, "I am healing. I am healing." Keep medi-

Practicing mindfulness
while you eat is good
for you, increasing
enjoyment.

tating on your healing mantra for a minute or two, or as
long as feels good. Then sit calmly for several seconds
as you again check in on yourself to assess your tension level after your healing meditation. How does your
after-meditating rating compare to the before rating? As
an alternative, rate your level of hope or level of expecting to get well before and after practicing your healing
meditation. Having a strong expectation that you will get
well builds hope, which has been shown to harness the
placebo effect, your body's power to self-heal.

Practice Mindfulness

MEDITATION DOESN'T HAVE TO BE limited to strictly defined
practice sessions: you can practice mindfulness during
your daily life. When stressed, for example, you might
take a few seconds to focus on your breathing, possibly thinking a mantra to empty your mind of negative
thoughts and the emotions they trigger.

Practicing mindfulness while you eat is good for
you, increasing enjoyment, and may even help you lose
weight. Focus first on the food and its arrangement on
the plate. Perhaps you can smell its aroma. Breathe it in
deeply. Place a bite in your mouth. Focus on the sensation of it being on your tongue—and then focus on
your chewing. Notice everything about the food in your
mouth—its taste, its texture. Sometimes there is a first
taste and then an after-taste. Search for that after-taste
and enhance it by giving it your total attention.

Living Mindfully

PERIODICALLY DURING THE DAY, stop and focus. Whether you are sitting at a computer, folding the laundry, or driving a car, become more aware of your body's movements and the feel of your clothing, for example. Notice the kinds of thoughts that go through your mind while you do this. Watch yourself objectively. Notice how you feel in the present moment. This is living mindfully.

Once you start to practice meditation, you will soon find yourself naturally gravitating to it in times of stress. This is a very effective way of communicating with the non-conscious part of your mind that controls your cells' response to their environment. External circumstances—stressors—may continue to push you toward the fight-or-flight response, which runs counter to your desire for health and wellness. Meditation will pull you in the opposite direction, helping move your body into balance, homeostasis—the state in which your cells can perform their naturally health-tropic functions and engage the placebo effect.

This can be a big step toward keeping yourself well and returning you to wellness when you become ill or are injured. And there are other steps that can move you even farther along the road to wellness. One of the most important is *visualizing*, which means seeing yourself—your body, your mind, your cells—in the state of health and wellness that you want to retain or to which you hope to return. Meditation can help open the door to visualization. And just as you can learn to practice meditation, you can learn ways to visualize the healthful state in which you want your body to function—as we will see.

14

See Yourself As Well

Y OU ARE CONSTANTLY RUSHING AROUND in your busy life, stretched and pulled in different directions by com- mitments to jobs, to family and friends. You are tense and pressured—stressed out! You know you need to unwind— but how?

Visualization is the technique of focusing your imag- ination on a mental image—a picture you create in your mind's eye. It can be used to relieve stress and refuel, to soothe pain, to accomplish goals like quitting smoking, and to heal yourself. Visualization is a form of self-hyp- nosis that anyone can use to improve health and perfor- mance. Athletes, such as runners improve performance by imagining running the course beforehand. Therapists have their clients use mental imagery to heal emotional pain, and experts lead visualization seminars to help peo- ple realize their dreams.

Visualizing a relaxing scene can lower blood pressure and levels of stress hormones in the blood and can be an adjunct to treatment of asthma, allergies, arthritis, can- cer, chronic fatigue syndrome, fibromyalgia, insomnia, chronic pain, and hypertension.

Envisioning

LEARNING TO ENVISION is similar to learning to speak. The ability to speak is an innate capability, but speaking itself must be learned. Forming the sounds and learning the meaning and syntax of language does not come naturally. You must work at it. We all have the ability to envision, but most of us haven't learned how to use this fantastic and uniquely (so far as we know) human tool. And worse, many of our teachers and schools suppressed, often unwittingly, our natural inclination to envision, calling it "daydreaming".

We all have an imagination, but most of us don't use it purposefully. Scientists have not been able to agree on where imagination actually occurs. But it helps to think of the back of your eyes or the inside of your forehead as a kind of mental viewing screen. Anything you can imagine can be projected onto your Mental Screen. You can sit back and observe the action or you can project yourself into the image, much as in a dream. But unlike dreams, which seem to come and go on their own, you can purposefully create pictures, try them on, see how they feel and rework them. The results can be powerful.

Study a Candle

ONE WAY TO BEGIN ENVISIONING is to observe an object for a length of time, then to close your eyes and picture the object in your mind. A burning candle works well—but you can use any object. Try studying a candle flame in

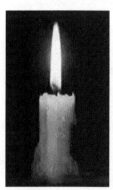

a darkened room. Sit in a comfortable position in front of the candle. Kick off your shoes and loosen any tight clothing. Dim the lights. Breathe slowly and deeply for two or three minutes to relax. Then study the burning candle. What does the flame look like? Notice how it flickers and flashes. Notice the color of the flame and how it changes when flickering.

Close your eyes while holding the image of the candle and flame in your mind's eye. Think of your mind's eye as a mental

Being in a relaxed state facilitates envisioning. Breathing slowly and deeply relaxes the body and mind.

viewing screen on the inside of your eyes and forehead. While continuing to breathe slowly, imagine that you see the burning candle on your viewing screen.

Open your eyes. Study the actual burning candle again, comparing it to your mental image. Watch how the flame flickers and flashes. Notice its many colors and how they become more intense when flickering.

Close your eyes and again project the image of the candle and flame onto your mental viewing screen. Compare the mental image of the flame to your memory of the actual flame. Add detail to your mental image.

The ability to envision varies. Some people "see" vivid pictures in color; others can't see anything. If this happens, just imagine what you *would* see if you *could* see the burning candle.

Walking on the Beach

CLOSE YOUR EYES while slowly breathing in and out. Using your Mental Screen, project the image of a beach on a beautiful day. The sky is clear blue, with the sun beaming down. Waves are lapping gently and the air is comfortably warm. Imagine that you are walking along the beach.

How did you experience imagining yourself walking on the beach? Did you watch yourself walking along the beach, as you would an actor on a movie screen? Or were you *inside your body* as you walked on the imagined beach, as you would be in a dream? Visualizing is less effective when you watch detached from afar. Instead, when envisioning yourself, always be "in" your body looking out. Noticing your senses puts you into your body into the visualization. Vision itself is only one sense. When you walk on a real beach you *see* the beach and the water, and you *hear, smell, feel,* even *taste,* being at the beach.

By imagining each sense and using it in the imaging, you can put yourself *into* the visualization—almost like stepping into a dream. So imagine walking on the beach again, and this time imagine experiencing each sense.

More Beach Walking

CLOSE YOUR EYES, while slowly breathing in and out. Using your Mental Screen, imagine walking on a beach on a beautiful day. This time be "in" your body. Imagine you are walking barefooted. How does the sand *feel?* Notice the *feel* of the sand between your toes. Notice the temperature of the sand and how it changes with each step. *Feel* a slight breeze as it brushes your hair across your forehead. *Hear* the lapping of the gentle waves. *Hear* the cries of the gulls, flying overhead. What do you *smell?* Smoke from a picnic fire? Is there a fishy smell? What do you *taste?* Salty air? *Feel* the warmth of the sun on the top of your head. *Feel* the tension in your leg muscles as you push your feet into the sand. *See* a boat off shore with gulls circling it. *Hear* a foghorn in the distance.

The more intense and real the image, the more powerful it is.

Visualization activates your body's ability to heal anything, from serious surgery to a sprained ankle.

—Jeffrey Rossman, PhD

Really *hear* the sounds in your imagination; really *smell* the smells in the vision. The more you use envisioning—or picturing—the better you will become at enlisting all of your senses to empower your visualization.

Use to Relax

BECAUSE WE HUMANS are so verbally oriented, we don't notice how much of our thinking is in images. With positive mental pictures and self-suggestion, visualization can change emotions, which have a physical effect on the body.

Imagining being in a pleasant scene, such as walking along a meandering stream or a forest path, is relaxing. Our bodies respond to the images in our mind as if they are real. So imagining yourself lying on the beach with the sun warming you, while listening to the lapping waves, can be as relaxing as actually being on a real beach. Vividly picturing a pleasant scene brings on the same positive emotions we would have if we were actually in the pleasant scene.

Create Your Pleasant Scene

PICK A SCENE you find pleasant for practice. You might be lying in your hammock on your deck. You might be sitting on a rock next to a babbling brook, watching the reeds waving and flowing in the water. Scenes don't have to be "real." You might be floating on a fluffy cloud or floating around the universe on invisible wings. That the scene is pleasant *for you* is what is important.

Close your eyes and imagine your pleasant scene— actually project yourself into the scene, as if in a dream. Notice what you see. Notice how it feels to be in the scene. What do you hear? Smell? Experience being in your pleasant scene for several seconds, noticing what comes into each of your senses.

What did you discover when you experienced your pleasant scene? Always make sure to engage all of your senses to make the pleasant scene as real and intense as you can. The more intense it is, the more powerful it will be in soothing you and relieving stress.

Using Your Pleasant Scene

GOING TO YOUR PLEASANT SCENE is a kind of self-hypnosis. The more you use the pleasant scene and feel relaxed while doing so, the more powerful it will become in putting you into a rejuvenated, relaxed state, which will nurture your cells, encouraging them to keep themselves well or heal themselves.

Your pleasant scene is a wonderful tool that you can use anywhere and at any time to relieve stress, relax and rejuvenate. You can kick back at your desk to regenerate yourself by "going to your pleasant scene" for a minute or two. Or suppose you ride a bus to work each morning. Instead of staring out the window at passing cars, you could imagine you were on an Africa safari, weaving in the sounds and bus movement. The imagination is a wonderful thing. *Use it often.*

Picture Healing Images

WITH POSITIVE PICTURES and self-suggestion, visualization can change emotions that subsequently have a physical effect on the body. Positive thought is essential to producing positive results. Negative thoughts and emotions lower the immune system, while positive thoughts and emotions actually boost immune functioning. Jose Silva, creator of the Silva Mind Control Method, believed that 90% of all illness is caused by the mind. If most illness is caused by the mind, then it is likely that most illness can be reversed by the mind.

Some physicians work with their patients to create healing visions to prepare them for the massive trauma of surgery. Here is an example of how Jerry Rossman, Ph.D., author of *The Mind-Body Mood Solution*, does this.

Amanda was worried about her upcoming surgery. Together, we designed the visualization experience. Then she closed her eyes and I guided her into a deeply relaxed state and suggested to Amanda that she see the caring surgical staff welcoming her. She imagined feeling relaxed and safe, knowing she was in good hands. I told her to imagine the team doing an excellent job, and to see herself handling the procedure well. Then I suggested she see herself recovering well after the surgery. I had her imagine the tissues of her body healing, knitting themselves together perfectly. I suggested that her body knows how to heal itself, and that she would support it with good nutrition, sleep, and relaxation. I made a recording of the 25-minute visualization, and Amanda listened to it every day at home.

Dr. O. Carl Simonton, a radiation oncologist and author of *The Healing Journey,* noticed that cancer patients who had a more positive attitude generally lived longer and had fewer side effects of treatment. When he added lifestyle counseling to medical treatment for patients with advanced cancer, their survival time doubled and their quality of life improved.

Simonton said that the course of a disease in general is affected by emotional stress. Simonton developed the first systematic emotional intervention used in treating cancer, and his program was approved by the surgeon general's office in 1973.

Many patients become discouraged and develop a feeling of helplessness and hopelessness, and this seems to go along with resistance to allow diseases to develop clinically. Often, for example, there is a loss. When people experience a severe loss, such as losing a child, some can adapt; others fall into a deep depression. It is not the loss but the person's negative response to the loss that can have an adverse impact on health.

Cancer patients have a tendency towards self-pity, which Simonton thinks is one of the most self-destructive aspects of the "cancer personality." Going along with it is a poor self-image with a limited capacity to trust oneself and other people. This can stem from rejection, real or imagined, that the patient has suffered . These patients have a strong tendency towards resentment, with a lot of difficulty in forgiving and letting go of perceived injustices. And many have a poor ability to develop and maintain long-term meaningful relationships.

"Your state of mind influences your health and it can influence the course of a person's disease"
— Dr. O. Carl Simonton

Healing Visions

SIMONTON ASKED CANCER PATIENTS to visualize their disease, to visualize their treatment and to visualize their body's immune mechanism. In one case a man said that his cancer looked like a big black rat and the treatment (which was chemotherapy and certain pills) going into his bloodstream like miniature yellow pills. Simonton asked, "What happens between the rat and the pills?" "Once in a while he eats one," the man replied. "What happens when he eats that pill?" Simonton asked. "Well, it makes him sick for a while and then he gets better again and fights me all the harder," the man answered. "What about your white blood cells and your immune mechanism?" Simonton asked. The man, who was a farmer, said "It looks like an incubator?" "What do you mean by incubator?" Simonton asked. The man answered, "You know, eggs are put into an incubator and a light shines down on them and then they hatch. One of these days my white blood cells will hatch." The way people picture their disease, their body's immune mechanism and their treatment gives many clues as to how they really feel about getting well.

Another of Simonton's patients was a young man who said he saw his cancer as a muddy, dirty lake and his white blood cells as a big white cloud that could cover the lake. Simonton asked, "How does the cloud get the cancer out of the lake?" The patient said that as long as the big white cloud covered up the lake he felt comfortable. So Simonton had him change his mental image and told him to picture something where the white blood cells were huge and more powerful than the cancer and there was a lot of action. So the patient pictured his cancer as a hamburger and his white blood cells as a giant polar bear eating up the burger.

One thing all these visualizations have in common—one thing that gives them all their power—is that the people picture what they want as existing in the here and now. That is, in the last example, the patient pictured his cancer as a

Before we can believe something will come about we have to picture it that way.

Picture what you want as existing in the here and now. hamburger and the polar bear eating it immediately—not at some point in the future. Before we can believe something will come about, we have to picture it that way—we have to treat it as if it is *already* coming about. This is a powerful way to engage the placebo effect.

How to Start

TAKE A FEW MINUTES to relax as deeply as you can. Breathe in slowly and breathe out slowly, while allowing yourself to relax. Each time you do this, you will relax even more easily and deeply.

With your eyes closed, imagine a movie screen in front of you—like the one in a movie theater. Project a picture of your current state of health on your mental screen. Make sure to include the ailment or pain you are experiencing. Actually *see* yourself in your current condition, on the screen. Your image doesn't have to be exactly the way your body looks. A lung, for example, can be a balloon; a kidney can be a kidney bean. Think of a picture for your ailment and feel the emotions associated with your health problem.

Now see yourself healing. See yourself getting better and healthier. Watch the ailment disappearing. Create with your imagination a system to remove the ailment. Kidney stones can be crushed into a powder and excreted. Joints can be oiled with an oil can. A tumor can be black blobs and white blood cells can be soldiers attacking it—and as it is attacked, imagine the tumor shrinking until it disappears. A sore muscle could be bathed in a healing light to alleviate pain. A broom can sweep sand out of an arthritic joint.

The exact image doesn't matter. The image of your ailment doesn't have to be scientifically correct. The image is metaphorical and symbolic. What matters is that what you create speaks to you. Your non-conscious mind works in images, symbols, metaphors and associations, not through logic and reason.

Now picture yourself in perfect health. Feel the joy and energy of being healthy. Imagine that it is really true. Trust your body's self-healing ability. *Believe* that healing is taking place. Understand that this visualization is an *aid* to medical treatment, not a substitute for it. You still need medical approaches, such as medications to suppress symptoms or relieve pain—because those medicines clear the way for your body to heal itself. So do not rely *entirely* on visualization and the placebo effect to make you healthy—but make visualization *part* of your arsenal of weapons to fight whatever ails you.

Visualization accelerates the mind's natural healing process. Visualizing is always done in the present tense. While you want something in the future, when visualizing you see yourself in that situation *in the now.* Never visualize "wanting" something; rather, visualize already "being" or having what you want. Picture what you want as existing

> "Your mind is in every cell of your body"
> —David Felten, PhD
> University of Rochester
> School of Medicine

in the here and now. Remember, before we can believe something will come about, we have to picture it that way.

A relaxed, meditative state puts your mind and body in a state that is conducive to healing, where stress is reduced and your immune system strengthened—and cells begin to repair and heal.

Mind Mirror

THE MIND MIRROR is another approach to effective visualization—remember that there is no one approach that is right for everyone. Try out several until you come up with one that works for you. To try this one, project a full-length mirror onto your mental screen. This is the mirror of your mind. Use this mirror to heal: look into the mind mirror and project an image of your current health condition into it. Study your condition. Study your appearance. Notice your expressions. Notice your posture. Notice your actions. Notice your attitude about your health. Really study and observe your physical condition.

Now take a deep breath. Erase the problem situation; have it simply disappear from the mirror. Project onto the mirror of your mind the healthy you that you desire to be. *See yourself in perfect health.* What are your expressions? How does a healthy you look? What are your actions? What do you do as a healthy you? What is your attitude? How do you take care of yourself? How do you keep yourself healthy? How is being healthy going to make your life better? See yourself perfectly healthy. Project intense desire to be healthy. Believe that you are becoming more and more healthy. Expect yourself to be healthy. See yourself as a healthy you.

When you are satisfied with the image of yourself as the perfectly healthy you, imagine stepping into the mirror—that is, imagine stepping into the healthy you reflected in the mirror. Experience feeling healthy, mentally and physically.

Beginning Visualization

VISUALIZATION IS A POWERFUL TOOL to engage the placebo effect, but one that many of us find we cannot use immediately and fully. If that is your feeling, begin with some short visualizations to become comfortable with the process. You can use a prepared guided visualization tape—search for one online; many are available. Or you can jump-start the process by attending a class; try searching for "visualization class" and your Zip code. Or you might have a few individual sessions with a coach—again, search for one online, or get recommendations from friends or healthcare professionals who have learned the power of visualization and support your use of it.

And remember to set the scene to make visualization easier for yourself. Try various approaches. You might experiment with soft music playing in the background. Burning incense can promote relaxation for some people, with a light aroma filling the air, engaging your senses to heighten your experience of deep relaxation. There are as many different forms of scene-setting as there are different approaches to visualization—and there is no right or wrong setting; just find one that works for you. The objective is to put yourself in physical circumstances that make it easier for you to produce the mental imagery of visualization in a way that will point your non-conscious mind in the direction in which you want it to go—the direction of health and well-being.

15

Appreciate

THERE IS AN ABUNDANCE OF THINGS for you to appreciate. For one thing, you are alive!! That is an awesome experience. Even if you do not live in an ideal location, even if you are not surrounded by people who support your health-oriented approach to life, even if your health is suboptimal and you are casting about for ways to heal yourself, there are many things to appreciate.

Finding Gratitude

EXPRESSING APPRECIATION can be a powerful way to promote self-healing. The fact is that feeling gratitude is good for your health; *expressing* it is even better! Studies have shown that expressing gratitude actually causes positive biochemical changes in your body, as well as improving your outlook in ways that are not measurable but are certainly real. Finding things for which you are grateful helps put your life and health in perspective, and to the extent that you realize you are much better off than some other people—even though your circumstances are not ideal—you create a positive mental framework to which your body responds at the cellular level with the placebo effect.

The reverse is true: if we feel *no* gratitude and believe we are beyond hope and in a situation that is awful in every way, our body responds to *that* at the cellular level and we end up feeling even worse—the nocebo effect.

It is true that "getting to gratitude" may take effort, because it requires a deliberate refocusing away from negative things and toward things for which you feel thankful. This means shifting focus away from the *don'ts* of life— what we don't have, what we want but cannot get, including material things and non-material ones—to what we *do* have and can be thankful for having. To be effective at the cellular level, expressions of gratitude need to be sincere, and getting to genuine thankfulness takes conscious purpose when everyday life provides so many pressures.

There is, however, something you can do—right now, this moment—to start toward thankfulness. Smile! It doesn't matter if you don't want to, if you feel you have "nothing to smile about." Do it anyway. Do not grimace— smile as genuinely as you can. If you need a "smile focus," find one in an everyday object near you. Look around you at the furniture and whatever might be on the walls, while noticing the colors. Think how much more wonderful life is in this world full of colors than it would be in one in black and white. Look at a paper clip and smile at the way it is twisted. Look out the window and perhaps you see a tree or bush. Smile in wonder at the way a leaf attaches to a branch. Look at this book and smile in wonder at the little squiggles and lines that make up letters that make up words that make up sentences—that you can read and understand!

Smile Often

SMILE AND SMILE OFTEN. Here's why. You know what usually makes you smile—a cartoon, a baby's expression, a puppy's bounciness, a movie or TV program. Experiencing these things causes your body to react, below the conscious level—non-consciously—by moving your facial muscles into the expression known as a smile. It also works in reverse! If you smile *even without having anything particular to smile about,* your body responds non-consciously with the same chemical and hormonal changes that normally *cause* you to smile. This is hard to believe until you try it and remarkable when you do. *Consciously* smiling creates the *non-conscious* body responses that normally *cause* you to smile—a smile gets you in tune with your body at the cellular level and actually makes you feel good, enhancing your health.

Think about it: earlier in this book, you experienced the reality that you could "operate" your body in specific ways with certain methods of breathing. Breathing is a tool for operating your body. So is smiling! You can operate your body in certain ways by smiling—whether you feel like smiling or not. Actually, after you smile, then you *do* feel like smiling!!!

Laughing is a related tool. There is a reason the phrase "laughter is the best medicine" has become a cliché. At the simplest level, when you are laughing you cannot also be feeling "down." So just as you can smile even when there is nothing particular to smile about, so you can laugh even when nothing particularly funny is going on. The effect is the same as with smiling: when you consciously bring into play the muscles that you normally use in laughter, you are signaling your body that there is something to laugh about—and your body produces the uplifting, health-promoting chemical and hormonal changes that normally *cause* the laugh. Your body simply associates a certain chemical and hormonal state with certain positions of facial muscles—so if you put the muscles in those positions, you get the positive, health-boosting effects of the cellular changes.

How does this tie to gratitude? Just as you can smile or laugh consciously rather than reactively to a stimulus, to operate your body in more healthful ways, so too you can turn your attention towards the abundance of plenty and beauty all around you, away from the *don'ts* of everyday life to the positive things for which you *can* be grateful. There are wonderful things you experience every single day. It may seem "natural" to focus on things you don't have—enough money, a good enough job, the right partner, the time to do all you want to do—but just as with consciously smiling, you can consciously turn your attention away from what isn't there to what is. And you can think seriously about how grateful you are for things that you usually take for granted.

Be Grateful For.....

• **Your health.** It may not be perfect, you may want to improve it, you may be seeking ways to stabilize it—but you can be grateful for what health you have.

• **Your family**—again, its members may not be perfect, but they are your relatives and provide a social connection and a blood-based inter-connectedness for which you can be grateful.

• **Your freedoms**—freedom of speech, thought, assembly, freedom to move where you want to, go where you wish, discuss and argue and invent and exercise your mind.

• **Your consciousness**— awareness of the world around you. Your intelligence and creativity.

• **Your memories**—positive or negative, they are an important part of who you are and in fact have helped make you who you are today.

• **The world outdoors**—all the wonders of sunshine, clouds, warmth, cold, rain, snow, ice, nature!

• **Your food**—you may not always have exactly what you want, but so many others have less, and you have access to a variety of foods that would be the envy of most people in the past and many people today.

• **Your work**—even if it is not exactly what you want, it gives you the income to do much of what you want to do on your own terms, to take advantage of the freedoms for which you are also grateful.

• **Your desire** to learn new things, an inquisitive spirit that can take you into areas you have not explored before, again furthering the freedoms you enjoy.

• **Your pets**—the animal companions who share your home and space and bring you warmth, unquestioning love, acceptance, as well as responsibilities that are different from family and work-related ones, making you a better-rounded person.

- **Your spiritual nature**—
the religious or philosophical system you believe in
and follow.

*Say what you want,
in your own words,
for just a minute a
day, out loud.*

As with the many little things at which you can smile, there are many small and not-so-small things for which you can be grateful. Do plants grow outside your home? Admire their shape and the magic of their color. Do you live in a city and grow small plants on the window sill? Admire the wonder of their "aliveness," the way they contrast with the hustle and bustle of life around you. In fact, be grateful for the sun that plants, indoor or outdoor, need to live—you need it to live, too, and can be grateful that it *will* come up tomorrow, the day after and the day after that.

Be thankful for your awesome mind—the mind that thinks problems through, overcomes adversity, even reads books to learn more about your health and ways to improve it! If you do not naturally have a habit of gratitude, you can create one by simply writing down things for which you are grateful whenever you think of them—call it a "What I Appreciate" or "What I Am Thankful For."

Add to your list regularly. Include the small things, like the smell of coffee when making breakfast. You might start off your work day by first reading over your Appreciation List. It will take only a minute or two to establish a productive mood. Notice and reflect on how good it feels to appreciate. This is what mystics mean when they say, "Stop to smell the roses."

Even beyond reading your list to yourself, *speak your gratitude.* "I am thankful for the birds I hear in the morning." "I am grateful for everything I learn from my children." "I am thankful that I have a job that lets me live in this house/apartment." "I am grateful for my health—and thankful that it is getting better." You are not talking to any person—you are making your feelings seem realer by saying them out loud, essentially asking your body, at the cellular level, to respond to your expression, just as it responds when you smile by making the chemical and hormonal changes that would normally cause the smile in the first place.

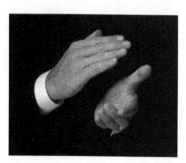

Attitude of Gratitude

STOP BEING SHY about your thankfulness. If you are standing in line in a local shop to buy an ice-cream cone, you might say to the person waiting next to you, "I love and appreciate ice cream. I'm looking forward to tasting it." Spread your appreciation around. This is how you create your own attitude of gratitude.

This attitude of gratitude will promote self-healing. Your mood will be brighter, your feelings more uplifted, when you realize all the things in your life for which you feel appreciation. Your life will feel more bountiful rather than filled with *don'ts*. You will have refocused—at least for part of the day, every day—on what is positive, on things you have and appreciate. And it is this refocusing that will help you heal yourself by inducing your body to alter its chemical balance and hormone production, at the cellular level, to preserve and boost your health.

Every type of energy you express, positive or negative, is reflected within you. If you express hatred or anger toward someone or something, an element of that expression affects you internally. You pay a price through the reflected negative energy you are bringing to bear through anger or hostility. By the same token, if you love someone or something—or express your thankfulness and appreciation toward a person or thing—some of the positive energy you direct outward remains within you. The act of expressing thankfulness and appreciation is itself a kind of self-healing.

Obviously it is not possible to be positive and upbeat about everything and everyone, all the time. Things do go wrong in life; problems occur; some people with whom we interact are unpleasant; some circumstances simply stink. And this is exactly why it is so important to take time every day, just a little time, to note things you appreciate and to speak your gratitude out loud.

Criticism and anger are at times useful. People who tell you that you should always be positive are simply being naïve. But anger—which comes with tension and tends to provoke a stress response that can make us feel worse after an initial outburst of "getting it off our chest"—cannot coexist with gratitude. The more time you spend finding things for which to be grateful, the more time you spend expressing your thankfulness, the less time there will be in your life for anger, hostility and other negative emotions that provoke the nocebo effect.

Expressing appreciation is self-reinforcing, especially if you find yourself thankful for everyday things rather than extraordinary circumstances. This is why it is important to list all the things, little as well as big, for which you are grateful.

Consider Charlene, who developed oropharyngeal cancer and underwent chemotherapy and radiation treatment that led to remission. As usually happens with this cancer, the therapy destroyed many of her taste buds, and the doctors said there was no way to know when or if they would grow back. Charlene decided to purposefully appreciate, during her recovery, things she could taste—even things that did not taste the same to her as they did before her illness. She started by being thankful for the sense of taste itself—and how many of us think about just how wonderful that is?

Although she became able to taste more things because her recovery was progressing, Charlene found that she could not taste certain things at all—and did not like the taste of some things that she used to enjoy. However, rather than resenting these losses, she focused on what she could appreciate about taste. She <u>did</u> like some things she had never before appreciated—milder foods than the spicy ones she used to favor, for example. She ate these foods slowly while savoring the tastes and thinking about how much she appreciated such pleasure.

Since Charlene, like all of us, needed to eat every day, she had many opportunities to feel gratitude for her ability to taste anything at all—and for her specific enjoyment of various foods whose taste she now found pleasant.

A Rock on a Path

YOU CAN EXPRESS GRATITUDE toward any thing or any person in the world and experience an increased ability to heal yourself—the choice is yours. There is something of a Buddhist experience about this: Buddhists will say that anything toward which you express thankfulness, even a rock on a path, will bring you measurable benefits if your gratitude is heartfelt and sincere.

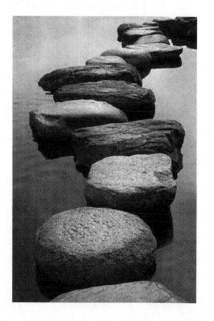

You can express thankfulness for life, for Mother Nature, for the universe or for God, and your gratitude will help instruct your body's cells to keep you well and restore you to health if anything disturbs your balance. The spiritual component need not be present, but if it is, it can give you a big boost toward self-healing. In fact, for many people it is one of the most important ways of all to encourage our bodies to heal themselves.

16

Optimism

LOWERING YOUR STRESS LEVEL—and therefore your body's production of stress hormones, which can suppress your immune system and leave you more vulnerable to illness—is a key part of healing yourself. And the positive thinking that typically comes with optimism is a key part of effective stress management and the many health benefits it brings.

Positive thinking does not mean you ignore problems. Rather, it means that you approach the unpleasantness in a more positive and productive way. You focus on the best that is likely to happen, not the worst. If the thoughts that run through your head are mostly negative, your outlook on life is more likely pessimistic. If your thoughts are mostly positive, you're likely an optimist.

Health benefits of positive thinking include:

- Increased lifespan
- Lower rates of depression
- Lower levels of distress
- Greater resistance to the common cold
- Better psychological and physical well-being
- Reduced risk of death from cardiovascular disease
- Better coping skills during times of stress

From a positive attitude, an attitude of optimism, comes hope—the feeling that things will get better, will work out fine, will emerge in the more-positive of two potential outcomes. Hope is crucial to engaging the placebo effect, since being hopeful of a positive outcome goes hand in hand with producing the bodily changes that signal your cells to behave in health-tropic ways.

Having a positive outlook enables you to cope better with stressful situations, which reduces their harmful health effects. One reason optimists may live longer is that it is thought that positive-thinking people tend to live more-healthful lifestyles: they get more physical activity and follow a more-healthful diet. If you can approach life in a more-positive way, you may find it easier to make changes that are known to be better for you in your overall lifestyle.

Think back to the last time you experienced a loss, setback, or hardship. Did you respond by venting, ruminating, and dwelling on the disappointment, or did you look for a faint flash of meaning through all of the darkness—a silver lining of some sort? How quickly did you bounce back—how resilient were you?

Far from being delusional or faith-based, having a positive outlook in difficult circumstances is not only an important predictor of resilience—how quickly people recover from adversity—but is also *the* most important predictor of it. People who are resilient tend to be more positive and optimistic compared to less-resilient folks; they are better able to regulate their emotions; and they are more able to maintain their optimism through the most trying circumstances.

James Pennebaker, a psychological researcher at the
University of Texas at Austin, has found that people who
find meaning in adversity are ultimately healthier in the
long run than those who do not.

Analyzing a writing exercise, Pennebaker noticed
that the people who benefited most from writing about a
negative experience were trying to derive meaning from
the trauma. They were probing the causes and conse-
quences of the adversity and, as a result, eventually grew
wiser about it. A year later, their medical records showed
that the meaning-seekers went to the doctor and hospital
fewer times than people in the control group, who wrote
about a non-traumatic event. People who used the exercise to vent, by contrast, received no health benefits.

Barbara Fredrickson, a psychological researcher
at the University of North Carolina at Chapel Hill, has
looked more closely at the relationship between being
positive and resilience and has found that having a
positive mood makes people more resilient physically.
Positive emotions can, researchers concluded, undo the
effects of a stressful negative experience. The researchers
found that the most resilient people were also more positive in day-to-day life.

With that in mind, the researchers wondered if they
could inject some positive attitudes into the non-resilient
people to make them more resilient. They primed both
types of people. The people who benefitted most from the
priming were non-resilient people. Those who were told
to approach a specific task as an opportunity rather than
a threat started looking more like resilient people in their
cardiovascular measures.

Resilient people also respond to adversity by appealing to a wider range of emotions. When your mind starts soaring, you notice more and more positive things. This unleashes an upward spiral of positive emotions that opens people up to new ways of thinking and seeing the world—to new ways forward. This is yet another reason why positive people are resilient. They see opportunities that negative-thinking people don't.

We have a choice in our perspective. We can focus on the positive or on the negative. But most of the time, we simply respond out of habit, not realizing that we are choosing our response. Your perspective has a powerful impact on your happiness and your health: it is easier to visualize being healed and healthy when you are optimistic.

So what if you tend to look on the down side and to be a worrier? What if your first tendency is to imagine the worst-case scenario? What can you do?

Optimism Exercise

IN THIS EXERCISE you will use a worrisome future event to study optimism and pessimism. The first step is to pick a worrisome event for practice. Maybe your pet is getting older and you are worried about its health and comfort. Maybe you have a limited income and you worry that your rent will be increased. Maybe your doctor did some lab tests and you are worried about the results.

After you have selected a worrisome event for practice, imagine the outcome you hope for and the outcome you fear. Write a description of each of these outcomes in a notebook or journal, leaving enough room to add more later.

Now make yourself comfortable, loosen any binding clothing, close your eyes, and take a slow, deep breath in, hold it for 10 or so seconds, then exhale and hold the empty feeling for about 10 seconds. Continue breathing slowly and deeply in this manner until you feel fully relaxed.

Crossroads

WHEN YOU FEEL RELAXED, picture in your imagination that you are standing at a crossroads, at the intersection of two winding roads that are moving further and further apart. Place the outcome you desire past the bend in one of the imaginary roads and place the outcome you fear past the bend on the other imaginary road. Picture yourself at the intersection of these two imaginary roads. Imagine looking down the road with the desired outcome around the bend. You can see some distance down the road. What do you see? Slowly look around. If you can't actually see anything in your mind, imagine what you would see if you could.

Now look down the road where the feared outcome is around the bend. What do you see down that road? How

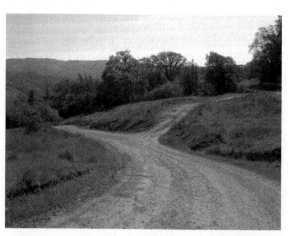

do the roads compare? What kind of roads are they? Dirt? Cobblestone? Cement? Tar? New? Old? What's alongside each road? Weeds?

Sidewalk? Trees? Buildings? Cars? What sounds do you hear? What is the light like? What else do you see? How do you feel as you look down each road?

In your mind, decide to follow the road to the outcome you hope for. Tell yourself: "I will follow my desires and dreams" as you imagine taking the first step on the road to your desired outcome. Notice how you feel as you take that first step. Now take another step and another as you proceed on the road to your desired outcome. What do you notice? Continue until you reach your desired outcome. Imagine being *in* the desired state. How do you feel?

Now come back to the present, here and now. Just sit for a few seconds, enjoying the relaxation and holding the feeling of being *in* your desired state. Return to the notebook where you wrote a description of your desired and feared outcomes, and jot down notes about what you saw in your imagination along the road to your desired outcome and how being there felt.

Repeat this exercise often as a way to retrain your thinking so instead of automatically going to the worst-case scenario, you train yourself to focus on what you desire the outcome to be. Remember that you are not ignoring the difficulties or worries inherent in a situation—you are accepting them, but are looking for something to occur other than the worst, most-pessimistic outcome. The more you do this, the easier it will become—and the better your health will be as your body produces fewer stress hormones as a result of your taking a more-positive view of the future.

17

Forgive

YOU HAVE MORE POWER TO ENGAGE your non-conscious mind in the task of keeping you well than you may realize. One of our most powerful weapons—one we do not use as much as we can, because we do not fully understand what it is—is *forgiving those who have disappointed and hurt you.* You can let go of past wrongs and your anger with the people who committed them, to free yourself from it. Resentment is a prison; forgiving your tormentor is the key to freedom.

We do not use this power as often as we might because, first, we do not realize how much resentment continue to cause us damage; and, second, because forgiving someone who has done us wrong feels like "giving in" to that person and "letting that person win." What we don't see is that this type of thinking is really a cover for our refusal to let it go, our refusal to stop resenting.

To forgive someone does not require you to communicate with that person at all—although that is certainly an option. Forgiving means you decide *for your own benefit* that holding onto anger and resentment—even fully justified anger and resentment—is doing *you* harm, and that giving up those feelings will give *you* benefit.

Emotional Disorder

THERE IS A SYNDROME called Post-Traumatic Embitterment Disorder (PTED) that can result from seething
bitterness and resentment building up on a daily basis
over a long period of time, according to a team of psycho-
therapists led by Prof. Dr. Michael Linden, professor of
psychiatry, psychosomatic medicine and psychotherapy
in the Charité University Hospital in Berlin. It is similar
and related to the better-known Post-Traumatic Stress
Disorder (PTSD) and can arise because of reaction to a
severe negative event, such as being laid off from a job
after years of sterling performance. This understandably
causes anger, resentment and bitter feelings.

Objectively speaking, losing a job—even a cherished
and lucrative one—is not in itself a life-threatening event.
But unresolved bitterness about the lost job can spawn
an array of serious illness-promoting problems such as
depression, insomnia, and serious emotional maladjust-
ment—symptoms of PTED. In extreme cases, people with
PTED may feel so let down that they lose their self-con-
fidence and their trust in others and even in former
friends, and may refuse to socialize, ultimately becoming
isolated. Their sense of being victims of injustice spirals
and becomes the con-
trolling factor in their
lives.

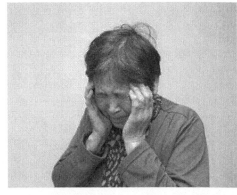

We do not have
to suffer a diagnos-
able condition such
as PTED to see how
holding onto hurts
and grudges, keeping

© chuugo - Fotolia.com

their anger and bitterness close within us, can affect us in highly negative ways. Bitterness, and the feelings of anger and depression that accompany it, may be linked to health issues such as cardiovascular problems and a weakened immune system. Ongoing bitterness may predict adverse changes in metabolism, immune-system function, and organ function. It can ruin the quality of your life.

It may be true that some difficulties in your current life are directly attributable to things that happened in the past. If, for example, you have a sibling who stole money from your parents' estate and used it as the foundation for his personal investments that you cannot afford to make because you did not receive what you were entitled to, then yes, you were wronged in a way that continues to affect you. But even in a case like this, the greater effect on you is not financial but health-related. By reviewing how you were wronged over and over in your mind, while telling yourself how your sibling betrayed you, you hold onto your anger and resentment. Whatever you think about becomes something that your non-conscious takes as "real," as happening now; and when it is something negative, such as being ripped off for your inheritance, your body triggers the stress response. So even though your sibling may have betrayed you fifteen years ago, your body—your cells—experience it as if it is happening *now*. This unrelenting bombardment with stress chemicals does damage and breakdowns result.

"Not forgiving is like drinking poison and expecting the other person to die."
—Nelson Mandela

Anger and embitterment hurt you, not your dishonest sibling, who is not stressed about the conflict, having forgotten it long ago. Instead, you pay a toll in your health and well-being for clinging to your resentment.

Psychologically, resentment refers to the mental process of repetitively replaying events that goad or anger us so that we re-experience and relive the events in ways that affect us emotionally, physiologically and spiritually to a very destructive degree. Ongoing resentment embodies a basic choice to refuse to forgive—an unwillingness to let bygones be bygones and bury the hatchet. We review and rehash our painful past by belaboring our resentments, imagining that we will somehow achieve the justice we believe we are due. We cling to a futile need to be right, to win, somehow, against the person who wronged us. Meanwhile, the person who wronged us is not distressed at all having long forgotten or stopped caring about the event we're belaboring needlessly.

Forgiving is your victory, not a victory for the person you forgive.

Clearly, resentment hurts you far more than the person toward whom you bear a grudge. Remember that it is you that is suffering by holding onto your anger and resentments inside of you. And this is where forgiving comes in. Forgiving is *your* victory, not a victory for the person you forgive. That person need never know you have forgiven him or her. The person may even be dead— many of us continue to carry around resentments of our parents long after they are gone. Forgiveness means *you* are making the choice to move beyond your past and get on with a better, more health-tropic life for yourself—the sort of victory embodied in the common saying, "Living well is the best revenge."

And, yes, you can forgive anything that has been done to you, if you *choose to do so*, because forgiving means to stop dwelling on it and to stop blaming and accusing. Physical injuries, sexual abuse and other traumas can stay with you throughout your life—it is a tall order to forgive anyone who perpetrates them, and it is presumptuous of anyone to say you "should" forgive them. Yet you do keep those abuses alive and able to continue to hurt you by the way that you think about those events. The decision to forgive rests entirely with you.

You have the option of practicing willful and deliberate *forgetfulness*—keeping in mind that these acts help *you* and do not constitute capitulation to the people you resent. Forgetfulness means teaching yourself to think of something else whenever an upsetting memory surfaces—letting the memory slide away into oblivion each time it emerges. This is akin to allowing intrusive thoughts about daily pressures to slide away from you when you meditate—you cannot stop the thoughts from entering your mind, but you can avoid dwelling on them. Forgiveness requires confronting the long-troubling thoughts and your memories of the person who did something bad to you—willful forgetfulness requires allowing the thoughts only brief entry into your mind, then letting them subside into the background as you focus on something else.

Let Go of Grudges

FORGIVING IS DIFFICULT, especially if you have been hurt or victimized severely, but both are tremendously beneficial for restoring your body to health and keeping it there. Remember to regard forgiveness as something you do for yourself, for the sake of your own health. This is the way to move closer to letting go of old anger and bitterness— which, however justified it may be, is holding you back from the health-tropic life you deserve.

Getting rid of grudges can reduce anxiety and lower blood pressure; in some people, forgiveness may even improve cardiovascular health. Only you can change your feeling and get rid of the burden of bitterness. Forgiving is not necessarily a "natural" thing to do: we are not born knowing how to forgive or even having a propensity to forgive. Forgiving is something we learn and get better and better at the more we do it. Like anything else worth learning, forgiving takes practice.

Forgiveness List

TRY THIS. Make a list of every person who has ever hurt you—including any you have forgiven already, because even in those cases, you may have lingering feelings of bitterness that you have not acknowledged. Review your list—and you can add people anytime—and rate, on a scale of 1 to 7, your level of hurt, resentment, upset or anger with this person, with 1 being very low and 7 being extremely high. Reorder the list from lowest to highest level of hurt and upset. This is your Hurt Hierarchy.

Start with the person with the lowest Hurt Rating. Imagine that person standing in front of you. Really try to "see" him or her in your mind's eye. If you can't actually picture the person, imagine how he or she would look and act if you could. Silently say to the person—or out loud if you want—"I forgive you (name) for (the transgression). I forgive you totally and completely. I release you and I release myself." Repeat this several times.

Really see the person in front of you when you do this. Imagine him or her as realistically as you can. The more intensely you can picture the person, the more effective your forgiveness will be *for you*. Remember, forgiveness is something you do for *yourself,* not for the person who hurt you—who, as in this exercise, need not be present and need never know what you have done. However, if you can tell the person—with sincerity—that you have forgiven him or her, then that is even more powerful.

Forgiveness Ritual

YOU CAN TURN FORGIVENESS into a portal for relaxation and even meditation, helping your body make a direct connection between your decision to let go of bitterness and grudges and your desire to live a more health-tropic life.

Sit quietly in a comfortable chair. Breathe slowly and deeply for one to two minutes as you settle into the chair, allowing yourself to relax. With your eyes closed, imagine a person you are angry at standing about five to ten feet in front of you. Breathe in and out slowly as you picture the person in as much detail as you can. Slowly draw your breath in through your nose, taking about one second or so. Hold it for a second, then slowly release your breath through your mouth. When you feel very relaxed from your controlled breathing, focus on the person who you are angry at standing in front of you—really see the person—as you continue your slow, deep breathing.

In your imagination, surround the person with whom you are angry with white light. Picture the person standing in front of you with a white, healing light all around. As you bathe the person in the white light, say silently, or out loud if you prefer, "I forgive you." To up the impact, see the person that you are angry with bathed in this white light, and mentally send your love—open your heart and send the person love while saying, "I forgive you."

After doing the ritual with a person who is high on your Hurt Hierarchy, you may still catch yourself being seduced into recounting his or her litany of sins. If you've spent years resenting what this person did, it will probably take a few forgiveness sessions to dissipate the hurt. We can hold grudges for years or decades, making it hard to eliminate them. Expect it to take more than one session for you to let go of the anger and resentment when the person has a high Hurt Rating.

When you catch yourself slipping into repeating the litany of sins, stop and remind yourself that your forgiveness is something you are doing for yourself and that it represents a victory for you and will promote the improved health and wellness you want. Willfully switch your thinking to something else—to something neutral or even pleasant to drive out your negative, resentful thoughts. It is even better, if you can switch to a positive thought about the person who hurt you. Repeat this forgiveness ritual as many times as it takes to forgive the person and let go of your anger. As you get more comfortable in subsequent practice sessions with forgiving the person, begin to send love and healing to him or her.

Move slowly through the people on your Forgiveness List. Don't rush. Remember that this is for you. The more you dispel your deep resentment, the greater the healing potential. Move through the people on the list from the lowest level of hurt to highest. Begin each session with a brief forgiveness "booster" with the one or two people you forgave previously. Then move to the next one on your list. Again, don't rush.

Practice Anywhere

ALTHOUGH THE FORGIVENESS RITUAL is most easily done in a quiet and comfortable place, you can actually practice forgiveness anywhere—in your car, at your desk, before going to sleep at night. In fact, forgiving before sleep can help you rest much more peacefully as your cells perform their health-tropic functions.

You can forgive people who are no longer here, or with whom you no longer have contact. Forgiving is about you and not the person being forgiven. That person could even no longer be living, such as a parent who has passed away. Death does not stop many of us from holding onto resentments. Sometimes it makes things worse, because there is no way to talk to that person—no closure. This may be the allure of mediums who say they can contact those who have passed on.

Forgiveness is not condoning the actions of the other person. It is not giving in or losing anything. Forgiveness frees *you* from a self-imposed prison, a *resentment prison*. And forgiving gets easier as you practice it more and more—and find yourself deriving the health-tropic benefits that result from forgiving and letting go of resentment.

18

Build Support

YOU ARE A SOCIAL BEING—we all are. Just as the trillions of cells in our bodies operate individually and
collectively to form the hive organism that each of us is,
so the billions of people on Earth function as individuals
but are also part of the collective of humanity. To some
people, this is a religious, spiritual or New Age revelation:
we are all connected. To some, it is a moral imperative,
as in John Donne's famous words in *Meditation 17*:

> *No man is an island, entire of itself; every man is a*
> *piece of the continent, a part of the main. If a clod be*
> *washed away by the sea, Europe is the less, as well*
> *as if a promontory were, as well as if a manor of*
> *thy friend's or of thine own were. Any man's death*
> *diminishes me, because I am involved in mankind;*
> *and therefore never send to know for whom the bell*
> *tolls; it tolls for thee.*

For our health, for our ability to harness the placebo
effect to stay well or return to wellness, what matters
in social interconnectedness is that we surround ourselves with people who will add to our health rather than
detract from it. We understand this intuitively when
we speak of, say, a "toxic" co-worker as someone to be
avoided, or a perpetual complainer as "bringing everyone
down."

One of the things we can do consciously to send messages into our non-conscious mind about the importance of maintaining and reinforcing health is to surround ourselves with people who have similar goals.

We humans are tribal animals. Our brains are not fully developed at birth—they, and our bodies, need protection to develop and grow, and this interdependence continues throughout life. Herd animals and animals that live in packs are similar: they need each other to survive and thrive. Whales isolated from their pods tend to die young; wolves isolated from their pack—lone wolves—are ostracized, left to fend for themselves and usually do not survive for long.

Health Benefits of Friends

HAVING CLOSE FRIENDS and family has far-reaching benefits for your health. A strong social support network can be critical to help you through the stress of tough times, whether you've had a bad day at work or a year filled with loss or chronic illness. Since your supportive family,

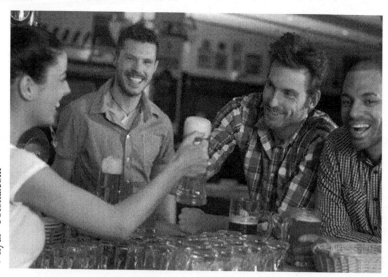

© nyul - Fotolia.com

friends, and co-workers are such an important part of your life, it's never too soon to cultivate these important relationships.

Numerous studies have demonstrated that having a network of supportive relationships contributes to psychological well-being. When you have a social support network, you benefit in the following ways:

- **Sense of belonging**. Spending time with people helps ward off loneliness. Whether it's other dog lovers, fishing buddies or neighbors, knowing you're not alone can go a long way toward coping with stress.

- **Increased sense of self-worth**. Having people who call you a friend reinforces the idea that you're a good person to be around. You are valued.

- **Feeling of security.** Your social network gives you access to information, advice, guidance and other types of assistance. It's comforting to know that you have people you can turn to in a time of need.

People who give off "positive vibes" where health is concerned tend to make you feel positive, too—while spending time around people with a negative outlook pushes you in the opposite direction. So to "persuade" your bodies to stay healthy and heal yourself if something does happen to disturb our homeostasis, it makes sense to surround yourself with people whose outlook on life and health is as positive as yours.

Living among healthy-minded, high-energy people who actively pursue health and happiness can lift your spirits, inspire you to make your own positive changes, and even give you examples of the health results you want to achieve. The difficult issue, though, is what to do with the people around you who do *not* have a positive attitude toward health. You may be able to avoid certain co-workers, but you can scarcely turn your back on friends—and more particularly on family—just because people live in ways that are not good for them.

This is where the nocebo effect comes in: being around health-oriented, positive people tends to encourage you in a positive direction, but being around negative people tends to push you the opposite way—making it harder for your body to marshal its forces to stay well and fight off threats to your well-being. It is all well and good for strangers to tell you that you should just get away from people who have a negative effect on you—but what if the person is a parent, a child, a longtime close friend, your spouse? It is all too common for a woman who is trying to, for example, eat more healthfully and exercise more regularly, to be confronted with the reality that her husband will not take up any physical activities and wants only to eat the meats and processed foods he is used to—few if any vegetables and no salads at all.

Reach Out

To improve your mental health and your ability to combat stress, surround yourself with at least a few good friends and confidants. Here are some ideas for building your social network:

- **Volunteer.** Pick a cause that's important to you and get involved. You're sure to meet others who share similar interests and values.

- **Join a gym or spa.** Or check out the local community center. Start a walking group at work or at your church. You'll make friends and get some exercise.

- **Take a class.** A local colleges and adult night school have many interesting and inexpensive classes. You'll meet people with similar interests.

Give and Take

A SUCCESSFUL RELATIONSHIP is a two-way street. The better a friend you are, the better your friends will be. A coffee break with a friend at work, a quick chat with a neighbor, a phone call to your sibling are ways to foster friendships. Don't wait for someone else to make the first move. If you meet someone interesting invite him or her to join you for coffee or another casual activity.

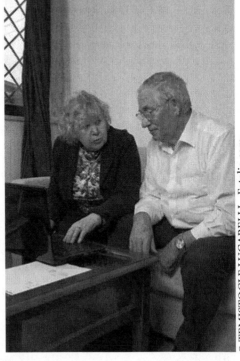

© TEMISTOCLE LUCARELLI - Fotolia.com

Suggestions for nurturing your relationships:

- **Keep in touch.** Answering phone calls, returning emails and reciprocating invitations let people know you care.

- **Be a good listener.** Find out what's important to your friends — you might find you have even more in common than you think.

- **Appreciate friends and family.** Take time to say thank you and express how important they are to you. Be there for them when they need support.

If you feel you just do not fit in with the people in the area where you now live—however you personally define "fitting in"—and if you are looking for the sort of supportive social environment that you can interact with regularly, with an eye toward keeping your body functioning optimally, then it may be worthwhile to consider living somewhere else. After all, the purpose of health-tropic living is to keep you happy, healthy and well-adjusted for the rest of your life. If you can connect with supportive people who, like you, want to help their bodies heal themselves and maintain health and homeostasis as much of the time as possible, then a geographical move may connect you with a supportive social structure that will make it all that much easier for you to pursue your own goal of enhanced health through the placebo effect. People have moved for worse reasons!

Taking the time to build a social support network is a wise investment not only in your mental well-being but also in your physical health and longevity. Research shows that those who enjoy high levels of social support stay healthier and live longer. So don't wait. Start making more friends or improving the relationships you already have. Whether you're the one getting the support or the one doling out the encouragement, you'll reap a plethora of rewards.

Watch for situations that seem to drain your energy. For example, avoid spending too much time with someone who is constantly negative and critical. Similarly, steer clear of people involved in unhealthy behaviors, such as alcohol or substance abuse, especially if you've struggled with addictions.

19

Pray

ONE REASON the medical establishment is uncomfortable with the placebo effect is that it works best when people *believe* it will work—and that gets into the thorny issue of belief itself, and thus of religion. This is not an area in which doctors are comfortable or one into which they wish to intrude. But an understanding of religion—or, more broadly, spirituality—is important to help engage the health-tropic nature of your body's cells.

Illness is not a punishment from God, but if you are ill and looking for ways to help your body heal itself—and if you are devout—then you may look to God for help in recovery. The appeal to something outside ourselves is an excellent focusing mechanism and can be a very effective way of helping our bodies get better and stay well. There is even evidence that prayer can benefit people who are not themselves praying. That is, if you and others pray for the recovery of someone else, that increases that person's chance of getting well. No, there is no absolute scientific proof of this, and skeptics will come up with reasons that it cannot be so, but in some studies, group prayer does seem to have helped to heal people who are distant from those doing the praying.

Prayer is a way of marshaling the body's innate wellness ability. Whether you believe that you reach out through prayer and touch God, or are touched by God, or that angels visit you and enfold you in their wings, or that something else—something unique to you—takes place, what matters is that prayer provides a focus point on something beyond your body and, if you are ill, beyond the illness. Many people talk about "faith healing" with a sneer, and that is the same sneer they reserve for the placebo effect—of which faith healing is one aspect.

But the placebo effect is real, and so, for some people under some circumstances, is faith healing. All of us have the power to optimize the body's chances of maintaining and recovering wellness on its own by changing our thoughts, beliefs, and feelings from negative to positive—which means, to the best of our ability, getting rid of hatred, resentment and anger, and choosing instead to fill our minds with relaxation, love and spiritual connection. This is what prayer does.

And sometimes prayer takes on aspects of the relaxation response, a form of mind/body connection in which we separate ourselves from everyday cares and pressures and allow them to flow through us harmlessly—while we get in touch with our inner selves and withdraw temporarily from the world so we can re-center and heal. If this sounds exactly like prayer to you, that makes sense, since in many ways it does resemble what happens when we pray.

The relaxation response is secular, but just think about how closely it resembles prayer.

Indeed, certain prayers call for almost exactly the same sort of inward—not outward—focus. The Catholic Rosary is a prime example. The Congregation for Divine Worship's directory of popular piety and the liturgy emphasizes the meditative aspects of the Rosary, calling it a contemplative prayer that requires "tranquility of rhythm or even a mental lingering which encourages the faithful to meditate on the mysteries of the Lord's life." And the structure of the Rosary itself makes contemplation all the easier. The sequence of prayers is the Lord's Prayer, the Hail Mary ten times, and the Glory Be to the Father—sometimes followed by the Fatima Prayer. Each sequence is known as a decade, and five decades are prayed—after starting with the Apostle's Creed and five initial prayers.

The Rosary involves repetition, which works much the same way that repetition of a word or sound does in eliciting the relaxation response. And there is a repetitious tactile element to the Rosary as well, with those who pray the Rosary holding each bead and repeating what is, in effect, a mantra. Catholicism requires that prating the Rosary be done in a very specific way, using very specific words, and to non-Catholics or nonbelievers in general, this may seem like a series of restrictions and strictures. But it has a purpose: to focus the mind and bring it into a state of inwardness and contemplation.

When the prayer is said repetitively in your mind, worries are blocked out. In fact, the praying of each decade is accompanied by meditation on one of the Mysteries of the Rosary, which recall the life of Jesus—there are currently twenty of them. So the idea is to use the repetitiveness of Rosary prayers to produce a sense of meditativeness that can be focused on Jesus. This is directly analogous to using repetitive sounds or phrases in order to produce a meditative state that can produce inward focus designed to maintain or improve health.

The reason prayer, meditation, the relaxation response and other forms of focus help elicit the placebo effect is that placebo activation is not a matter of the conscious mind. You cannot "think yourself well," because the process does not use the conscious mind. *Cells know how to heal themselves, but must be given the opportunity.* The brain may use only 40 watts of electricity, but it does a huge amount with a small helping of power, and this *is* electric power—intertwined with chemical signals that tell cells what to do and help the cells figure out what is going on around them so they can support or counter it.

Prayer Groups

IF THE USE OF PRAYER to get in touch with your non-conscious mind and health-tropic cells is appealing to you, consider forming a prayer group. Group prayer was a characteristic of the early Christians, and there are also many references to group prayer in the Old Testament. Make your group prayer experience inspirational and enjoyable so you and others leave refreshed and renewed. It is important to pick an element to structure the meeting around, enhancing the sense of community that comes when people meet for a common purpose and to communicate with God at the same time.

Meeting Elements

THE GROUP SHOULD HAVE A LEADER—a position that can rotate at each meeting. The leader introduces a prayer request, then allows the group a few minutes to pray for it. Then the leader introduces another request. Designate someone to close at the end of each prayer time to help ensure the group meeting does not go on too long. For purposes of engaging your health-tropic cells, you can mix thanks to God with requests for enhanced wellness, as in these examples:

- Thank God for your wellness.

- Thank God for something that happened in your life today.

- Ask God to help you or someone else with a health issue.

- Thank God for answering your requests.

An alternative approach is to pray using Scripture. Select a passage of Scripture as a guide for praying. For example, someone might read a Psalm of praise, such as Psalm 103, then pray a simple prayer relating to that verse. Other members should voice agreement or agree silently. Then the next person may follow with a different prayer—Psalm 145, for example—and others follow with their prayers.

The first person reads a phrase or verse aloud, then prays a simple prayer relating to the phrase or scripture verse. Other members of the group join in audibly or silently agree. The next person reads a different verse, then pauses to pray aloud. Others follow with their prayers.

For eliciting the placebo response, some people find that prayers of praise work best; others look for elements of Scripture showing how God eventually helps those in turmoil provided that they show and maintain their belief—as in, for example, the book of Job.

There are two other elements that prayer groups may find useful in seeking a focus on health and wellness:

Thanksgiving: Give thanks to God for who He is, what He has done, what He will do in our lives and what He is doing in the ministry—this is a prayer of gratitude.

Supplication: Ask God for His divine help to meet needs, solve problems, work in someone's life, and lead the group in supplication by praying aloud.

A popular alternative for group members who cannot meet is to agree to pray at the same time each day. This way, although not all members are in the same location, each member can feel spiritually connected to the others while praying. We do not really know a way to be sure of harnessing the power, electrical or otherwise, of *multiple* brains, but certainly the prayer of numerous people—all directed at a specific goal, such as the healing of someone who is not in the prayer group—has *some* electrical effect; *some* signal goes out to the Universe.

Exactly how it does so is not known; whether direct divine intervention takes place, or whether there is a Kirlian aura or an angelic response or some potent alteration in a Universal force, is unproven and perhaps unprovable. But there is nothing wrong with calling spontaneous self-healing—a universally acknowledged phenomenon—a miracle. Doctors use the word themselves. The fact that it does not occur *all* the time should not make us be less in awe of the fact that it *does* occur *some* of the time.

Prayer causes brain changes. But prayer within a structured religious context is not the only spiritual connection that can help us produce the placebo effect. Meditation, which may or may not have a strongly religious connection, has profound effects as well. It is another way to elicit the relaxation response. Andrew Newberg, M.D., a neuroscientist at the University of Pennsylvania, former director of the university's Center for Spirituality and the Mind, and author of *How God Changes Your Brain,* has commented, "The more you focus on something—whether that's math or auto racing or football or God—the more that becomes your reality, the more it becomes written into the neural connections of your brain."

It is the focus that is crucial—prayer is essentially a mechanism for focusing on your relationship with God, but if you have a strong relationship instead with, say, Nature, then finding ways to promote *that* focus will bring your body the same benefits that adherents of traditional religions obtain from prayer.

Prayer is only one route, albeit a very powerful one, toward maintaining and enhancing physical wellness. For example, John E. Welshons, author of *When Prayers Aren't Answered,* has commented, "There are two primary methods available to us for establishing an inner dialogue with God. They are prayer and meditation. Prayer can be defined as 'talking to God.' Meditation can be defined as 'listening to God.' It is a simple but profound distinction."

Increasingly, medical and academic institutions are studying the physical effects of prayer, meditation and other forms of intense mental focus. It is becoming more common to find spirituality research centers in university medical schools, such as the Duke Center for Spirituality, Theology and Health at Duke University. And prayer is getting attention in peer-reviewed medical literature.

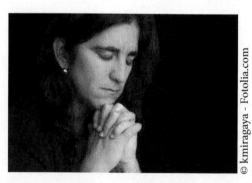

As early as 1999, William R. Miller and colleagues, in an article for the American Psychological Association called "Spirituality and Health,"

© kmiragaya - Fotolia.com

observed that "spiritual and religious involvement is not only common but is often important in clients' lives and has been generally linked to positive health outcomes. ... Incorporating spiritual perspectives in secular treatment has been found to improve outcomes for religiously oriented clients."

In *The Anatomy of Hope: How People Prevail in the Face of Illness,* Jerome Groopman, M.D., wrote, "Researchers are learning that a change in mind-set has the power to alter neurochemistry. Belief and expectation—the key elements of hope—can block pain by releasing the brain's endorphins and enkephalins, mimicking the effects of morphine. In some cases, hope can also have important effects on fundamental physiological processes like respiration, circulation and motor function. During the course of an illness, hope can be imagined as a domino effect, a chain reaction in which each link makes improvement more likely. It changes us profoundly in spirit and in body."

Wellness

YEAR AFTER YEAR, the evidence increasingly shows prayer and meditation—and more-secular forms of intense mental focus—as significant contributors to wellness, to the placebo effect under which our bodies maintain health and restore themselves to it when under attack by illness or injury. We can and should pray if that is our method of reaching out, reaching beyond ourselves, and finding focus and comfort that we are not alone. If you do not pray in accordance with the Catholic Rosary or other traditional forms of communication with the divine, find a way to make connections beyond yourself in whatever manner works for you. This reaching out has been known to religious and spiritual communities for thousands of years, which shows that science sometimes fails to keep up with what non-scientific groups learn and practice first.

Science does not have all the answers, and although it continues to find more of them every day, there are some that may remain forever beyond its capabilities. And even if they do not—even if science one day solves the puzzle of how prayer and meditation can help keep us well and restore us to health—the wonders of these self-guided approaches will not be diminished in the least.

Eileen E. Morrison was somewhat over-optimistic when she wrote in *Crucial Issues for the 21st Century,* "Over the past two decades a transition has been occurring in the healthcare industry; people are starting to express an interest in healing again. Of course, when we are discussing healing we are referring to it with its old English derivative, 'the making whole,' acknowledging that healing cannot occur without recognizing it as a spiritual process. Because of this renewed interest, attitudes toward spirituality in the [medical] workplace appear to be changing...a transition to a deeper calling is becoming apparent."

Science does not have all the answers.

But Morrison was correct in observing that, increasingly, "research suggests that patients desire and feel more comfortable with physicians who are not only open to their own humanity, but who also are willing to allow patients to discuss their spiritual proclivities." And all of us need to *practice* our spiritual proclivities as well, not just talk about them. They are a powerful method of healing ourselves.

20

Laugh Often

REMEMBER THAT EXHAUSTED FEELING after a good laugh—where your eyes water, you can't catch your breath, your side hurts, and your body is totally spent? It feels as if you've just finished a two-hour session at the gym. Laughter and exercise have much in common—most notably, both can boost your health.

Laughter really is the best medicine. It lowers blood pressure. People who lower their blood pressure reduce the risk of strokes and heart attacks. Laughing reduces stress hormone levels, which cuts the anxiety and stress affecting your body. Additionally, the reduction of stress hormones promotes higher immune system performance. Laughing along as a friend tells a joke can relieve some of the day's stress and help you reap the health benefits of laughter.

Laughter helps tone your abs. When you are laughing, your stomach muscles expand and contract, similar to when you exercise your abs. Meanwhile, the muscles you are not using to laugh are getting an opportunity to relax. Laughter is a great cardio workout. It gets your heart pumping and burns as many calories per hour as walking at a slow to moderate pace.

According to researchers, laughing 100 times is equivalent to 10 minutes on a rowing machine or 15 minutes on a stationary bicycle. But you don't need to break a sweat in order to have a really good laugh. Laughter momentarily clears the respiratory system. Just as with exercise, people tend to take deep breaths in and out during heavy laughter, which helps unclog airways and enhances inhalation and oxygen intake.

Laughing boosts T cells. T cells are specialized immune system cells waiting for activation. When you laugh, you activate T cells that immediately begin to fight off sickness. Laughing triggers the release of endorphins. Endorphins are natural pain killers. When laughing, your body produces endorphins, which ease chronic pain so you feel good all over. Laughing produces a general sense of well-being.

Laughter is one of the best natural pain relievers around. It's effective, free and available everywhere without a prescription!

Laughter eases fear and anger, allowing us to deal better with reversals. Laughter is a perfect distraction when dealing with a painful situation. The good feelings triggered by laughter may stick around a little longer, even after the pain has subsided. Doctors have found that people who have a positive outlook on life tend to fight diseases better than people who tend to be more negative.

Laughing decreases stress. When you roll on the floor in hysterics, stress melts. Levels of stress hormones such as cortisol and epinephrine, which suppress the immune system, tend to decrease during bouts of laughter. These hormones open the way to a host of infections, illnesses and general poor health. One study found that laughter helped reduce stress and improve immune function—or natural killer (NK) cell activity—an indication that laughter may be a beneficial addition to treatments for cancer and HIV patients. NK cells are a type of white blood cell that attacks tumor cells and those infected with a virus. Physical and emotional stress upset the balance of prolactin, insulin, thyroid and other hormones.

So the next time you're feeling stressed after reading about what's going on in the world, flip the newspaper to the comics and lighten your mood. Laughter has been shown to lower or balance blood pressure and increase vascular blood flow. By reviving blood circulation and increasing oxygenation of the blood, laughter may be a powerful ally in the fight against heart disease. Heart disease may not seem like a laughing matter, but laughter is a great addition to treatment. Blood pressure and circulation benefit from a hearty sense of humor, and your body will experience a boost of aerobic activity each time you chortle.

Results from a University of Maryland study linking laughter to cardiovascular health indicated that laughter seemed to cause the endothelium, tissue that composes the lining of blood vessels, to expand, allowing for better blood flow. It's crucial to pay attention to these cells because the endothelium plays an important part in the fight against atherosclerosis (thickening of the arteries),

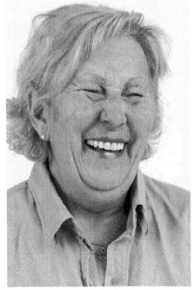

No one is suggesting that heart disease patients should use comedy clubs in lieu of medication, but laughter can have some astounding therapeutic results on cardiovascular health. Finding something to laugh about may help a patient's heart as well as his soul.

Laughing also affects blood sugar levels. Researchers think that laughter affects the neuroendocrine system and restrains blood sugar levels from spiking, or it may cause the acceleration of glucose use by muscle motion. Another study tracked the effect of long-term laughter therapy on the renin-angiotensin system, which regulates blood pressure, in subjects with type 2 diabetes. Most notably, plasma renin levels dropped dramatically, an indicator that laughter may help diabetics avoid microvascular-related complications.

Anatomy of an Illness

NORMAN COUSINS, who suffered from a painful, debilitating disease, found that using laughter as part of his treatment offered relief—even though temporary—from his crippling symptoms. He published these observations in his autobiography, *Anatomy of an Illness*.

Laughter is the knife that cuts tension from a room, allowing everyone to relax. When laughing, we become calmer and less aggressive, which help us develop "perspective" about what's going on. Releasing negative emotions, such as aggression, fear and anger, through laughter, provides psychological benefits. Laughter relaxes muscles, which reduces stress and offers relief for people dealing with spasm-related muscle pain.

Laughter energizes organs and improves blood flow, suppresses stress hormones and gives you a burst of exercise. In other words, laughter sends a wake-up call to the heart, brain and lungs and stimulates these organs into action. Laughter is even believed to aid in digestion. Some "laughter yoga" enthusiasts believe this type of therapy can help with symptoms related to conditions such as irritable bowel syndrome and diverticulosis.

Laughter boosts the immune system, decreasing stress hormones, improving circulation and oxygen intake. When laughing, you can barely catch your breath because of chuckling, even snorting—eventually coughing or hiccupping, which helps to loosen mucus and clear airways.

Incompatibility

ANOTHER THING ABOUT LAUGHING is a phenomenon that psychologists call "incompatibility." You can be tense or you can be relaxed, but you can't be tense and relaxed simultaneously, because the two conditions are incompatible. One strategy for reducing tension is to deliberately engage in an incompatible action—such as relaxing, for example. Laughter and tension are also incompatible. We've all been in a tense situation where someone made a joke or burst out laughing and the tension was released, making it easier for everyone to get on with the task at hand.

A Humor Perspective

FINDING THE HUMOR IN A CRISIS takes looking at it in a different way and appreciating the absurd. When worrying, you get stuck in one fixed view, which you take very seriously. You read the situation as a threat, which mobilizes the stress response. To find humor in a tense situation, step back and look from a new perspective to see it as

absurd. Once you've considered the situation as absurd
you have broken its grip and lessened the seriousness of
the dilemma. When you stop worrying and "awfulizing"
with all of its extreme negativity—even for a few minutes—you give yourself a few moments of relief from the
unrelenting tension that accompanies worry.

Finding humor in a situation is not something you
are born with. It is a way of looking at and thinking
about situations and difficulties. A sense of humor is a
set of specific, learned skills. Like any other skill, it must
be practiced—exercised, just like exercising your biceps
to keep them in shape. You need to exercise your sense
of humor to keep it in shape for times of stress, when
you really need it. Looking for what's funny in tense
situations will help you thrive in change, remain creative
under pressure, work more effectively, play more enthu-
siastically, and stay healthier in the process. You will be
more relaxed dealing with stressful situations and more
flexible in your approach. When you ruminate, you get
stuck in one rigid and generally ineffective approach.
Use humor to uncover a fresh perspective and boot your
thoughts on to problem solving.

Practice Smiling and Laughing

AS WE HAVE SEEN, when you smile you send a message
to your emotional brain that there must be something
funny happening. This primes the pump, so to speak.
Remember the old saying, "smile and the whole world
smiles with you"? When you smile you raise your spirits
and those of people around you. When you smile you
worry less. Things don't seem as catastrophic. To a certain degree, you can actually generate positive feelings
simply by the act of smiling.

Smile Exercise

ASSUME A COMFORTABLE SITTING POSITION. Count to three and, on three, take a deep breath, quickly stand up and smile the biggest smile that you can smile. Make sure that your teeth show. Sit back down and repeat the exercise several times. The fun of this exercise can be increased by doing it regularly with your family or co-workers at the office. When you feel tension coming on, take a deep breath, stand up, and smile broadly several times.

Watch Funny Movies

NORMAN COUSINS' INCURABLE CANCER was anything but funny. He suffered *ankylosing spondylitis*, a disease that destroys the connective tissue holding the spine together. At the low point of his illness he could barely move his arms and legs to turn over in bed and his jaw was almost locked. Remembering reading about the detrimental effects of negative emotion on the body, he wondered if positive emotions would produce positive chemical changes. That's when he got the idea to systematically give himself massive doses of humor.

Cousins watched funny movies. He made the discovery that 10 minutes of genuine belly laughter had an anesthetic effect and enabled him to get a couple of hours of pain-free sleep. Cousins later scientifically affirmed the power of laughter. He had sedimentation-rate readings done just before, as well as several hours after a laughing episode, and each time there was a small drop in the rate after laughter. Other research has substantiated the positive power of laughter. One study conducted by researchers from Cornell University showed that after seeing a funny movie, people demonstrated more creative flexibility, whereas people who did not see the funny movie suffered from "functional fixedness" on problem assignments.

Develop a Joy List

A DISCIPLINED JOY IN LIVING is a humor skill that allows those who possess it to draw strength from circumstances that would defeat other people. You can choose the way you look at things. You can look at the glass of water and complain that it is half empty. Or you can choose to look at things as challenges and opportunities. You can rejoice that the glass is still half full. It may not feel as if you're making a choice to worry when caught up in a major worrying bout, because it is so habitual. Worrying, which is dosing yourself in the nocebo, has become automatic as the impulses flash along those well-worn neural pathways.

The key here is disciplined joy in living. Discipline has many meanings, among which is to bring to order and obedience by training and control. It won't happen spontaneously; you must train your mind. The joy list is a helpful tool. A joy list is simply that: a list of activities and situations that bring *you* joy.

The tragic thing is that many people can think of only a few joyful things. Their lives have become so serious, dominated by responsibilities and worries, that they've lost their sense of joy. For too many, life is a long path of work and drudgery, with little fun or joy.

A Joy List is a great tool for helping you rediscover your joy. Carry a pocket-sized notebook. Or try file cards rubber-banded together for exercises like this. Use the notebook or file cards to compile a list of joyful things. Joy is an emotion of delight and happiness caused by something good or satisfying. It is a source of pleasure. Note in your pad or on your cards anything that makes you smile, laugh or feel good. Joyous activities might include taking your dog to the local dog park for an off-leash run with dog friends, browsing dusty books in an antiquarian bookstore, going to a drive-in movie with your spouse, calling a friend on the phone, or surfing the Internet and finding a new, exciting Web site. The possibilities are endless.

Joyous activities don't have to be stupendous events. They are *moments* of delight, ones that leave you simply feeling good, feeling alive. Especially important are the small things, the brief moments of joy. The refreshing feeling of a breeze on your cheek on a hot summer day, the aroma of your favorite pot roast cooking for dinner, the silkily sensuous feeling of your cat's fur as you pet it, are small things that add to the quality of life, bringing a joy in living—if you're paying attention.

Schedule Joy

IF YOU WANT MORE JOY in living, schedule joyful activities onto your calendar—especially on weekends. Don't let your weekends and evenings just happen. Be disciplined—systematically schedule fun into your life. Review your joy list and make sure that, to start, you schedule at least one joy-provoking activity each weekend day, including Fridays. Then build from there.

Remember that you can choose to feel happy and joyful or you can choose to sit around feeling worried and lonely. Worry may seem automatic and natural, while doing joyful things may feel forced and artificial. But that is because worrying is a well-worn bad habit. With discipline and practice, feeling a joy in living can become natural, too. Now, take a deep breath, stand up and smile the biggest smile you can.

21

Listen to Music

MUSIC HAS REMARKABLE MOOD-ALTERING POWER: you can change your mood faster with music than by taking drugs. One minute you're in a funk and the next minute you are tapping your foot to an upbeat, jazzy tune. Most of us have experienced this. By listening to music you can calm down, reduce stress and anxiety, lower blood pressure, and reduce the intensity of pain. Food can even be tastier: University of Minnesota researchers showed that singing "Happy Birthday" before eating a slice of cake actually made the cake taste better.

Listening to a half hour of soothing music each day can lower your blood pressure, according to research presented by the American Society of Hypertension, because slow instrumentals promote a sense of calm. Researchers from Finland showed that listening to music even helped to improve verbal memory in stroke victims.

Health workers use music for many conditions. It eases anxiety in cancer patients, and during surgery on patients with Parkinson's disease, certain types of music were found to provide significant comfort. Joyful music is linked with dilation of the inner lining of blood vessels, which means blood flows better and the heart stays healthier. Anxiety-prone people who listen to music are less likely to feel pain, and kids who take music lessons are better able to recall words—while older people with musical training have better mental sharpness than others of the same age, and people who suffer a stroke recover better if they listen to music soon afterwards.

Music is also used in connection with Tourette's syndrome, Huntington's disease, brain injury and Alzheimer's disease: the American Music Therapy Association says music soothes anxiety, pain, and depression, and lowers blood pressure. Listening to music accelerates healing and increases social interaction.

Listening to music is an easy way to slow down and get in touch with your body. It is not intellectual, which is a matter of words and talking to yourself; instead it is feeling and moving—it is repetition and rhythm. Research out of the Utah Pain Research Center found that listening to music aided anxiety-prone people in reducing feelings of pain. For some people, music can be as good in reducing anxiety as an actual physical massage.

Listening to music is an easy way to slow down and get in touch with your body

Self-Tuning

MOVING WITH MUSIC involves a kind of resonating—call it Self-Tuning. This means feeling the music's effects on you, really experiencing the tunes, rhythms, tempo changes, instrumentation, dynamics, pacing—the ways in which the music stays the same throughout, the ways in which it changes, and the ways your body responds when it does. We will explain this in more detail when discussing how to make your own playlists for specific purposes. For now, just realize that music can serve many purposes for your body.

Soothing music moves your mental focus inward, offering a way to reach into your body and down to your cells to harness the placebo effect. Upbeat music engages the placebo effect in a different way, encouraging your body to "pep itself up" to adjust its rhythms to those of the music. For example, University of Maryland Medical Center research showed that listening to joyful music is linked with dilation of blood vessels, causing improved blood flow.

Contemporary composers, such as Marc Neikrug, incorporate soothing elements in some works for the express purpose of encouraging healing and wellness. About his orchestral piece, *Healing Ceremony*, Neikrug says, "I thought about the power music has over people; I wanted to write something that would change how your body feels—helping you calm down, handle stress, get in touch with inner feelings and inner thoughts."

Classical music is an especially powerful way to tap into your innate ability to heal yourself. A normal resting heart rate for adults is from 60 to 100 beats per minute. Much of classical music ranges between 60 beats per minute and 140 beats per minute—which simulates the rhythm of your heartbeat and can induce relaxation, causing tranquility in the body. A Japanese study reports that people prefer music with a tempo in the 70 to 100 beats-per-minute range. This range is congruent with human heart rate during normal everyday situations.

By the same token, music can be used to increase your heart rate deliberately—especially useful for exercise. For that purpose, the tempo should be 120 to 140 beats per minute, or even 150 for intense exercise.

Music causes a level of arousal directly proportional to its tempo. And the music's speed is only part of what gives it its effect. Crescendo—that is, gradual volume increase—in music increases heart rate and respiration as well.

Just as music can speed heart rate and help "pump you up" for exercise or intense activity, listening to music that is slow or meditative in tempo decreases heart rate and slows breathing. Such music has a generally relaxing effect on the body. Decrescendo—or gradual volume decrease—in music dilates blood vessels during listening, causing a decrease in heart rate. Silence and respites in music create the same effect in heart rate.

To sum up: a person's heart rate changes while listening to music, and whether the heart beats faster or slower depends on the tempo of the music and other factors, such as whether the music gets gradually louder or softer.

New technological advances can actually make it possible to match your music library to your heart rate. MP3 players that act as a heart-rate monitor and pedometer as well as a music player can automatically select music to complement your heart rate. Consumers are required to program in selections they think will help them achieve their fitness goals; the selected songs will play as the consumer reaches the target heart rate.

But these will not necessarily be songs you would have chosen for yourself—you may not care for the performers or for the form of the songs, such as whether they are vocal or instrumental. So instead of looking exclusively to technology to provide the benefits of music, you can look to yourself—your body's own responses—by creating playlists specifically designed *by you* to accomplish what you want music to do.

Tailor Your Playlists

BY PAYING ATTENTION to music's effects on your body,
you can make personal playlists that reflect your own
musical tastes and that also reach down to your body
at the cellular level to engage your cells' health-tropic tendencies. You can make as many playlists as you
like. To start with, consider making a *soothing playlist*, a
mood-boosting playlist and a *workout playlist*.

Start by Self-Tuning your soothing playlist. Many
times in this book you have rated yourself on a scale for
tension or other feelings before and after experimenting
on yourself with various exercises. Use this same process
to sort through music to pick out songs that are good
for you—songs you can use to manage your moods and
manage your tension.

Pick a time and place when you'll not be distracted.
Select four or five songs that you know and think of as
soothing—best to start with instrumentals so as to not
be distracted by words. Get comfortable—sit in a comfy
chair, on pillows, on a comfortable couch, on a big pillow
on the floor, or anywhere that you find relaxing. Wear
loose-fitting comfortable clothing.

Before listening to any music, study how you feel
right here, right now. Notice your level of tension. Observe your tension for a few seconds and then rate it on a
scale of 1 to 9, with 1 being very low tension and 9 being
extremely high tension.

Now listen to your first soothing song for a minute or
so. Do not analyze it or think about it at all—just listen, letting your mind flow along, noticing the tune, the
rhythm, whether the music gets louder or softer, whether

it speeds up or slows down, what instruments are play-ing. Simply tune yourself into the progress of the music, letting it carry you along at its pace, with its rhythms, sounds, instrumentation and speed. This is Self-Tuning.

After a minute or two, stop and rate your tension level again on the scale of 1 to 9 you used at the start. If your tension level went down, then consider this song as a possible addition to your soothing playlist. (If it stayed the same or went up, move on to the next song.)

Now, play the song again, and this time—while you notice the tune, rhythm, speed and instruments of the songs—try consciously to match your breathing to the beat. As the song goes faster, breathe more quickly. As it slows down, breathe more slowly. When it stays at the same pace for some time, consciously breathe at that speed along with the music. Continue matching your breathing to the song for a minute or two, or even longer. Then stop and once again rate your tension level on the same scale of 1 to 9 you have been using. If your tension level has dropped further, then keep this song: it is now part of your soothing playlist.

For example, suppose you had a rough day at work and, even when you get comfortable and sit in a cozy chair, you find yourself with a high tension level of, say, 8. Then you listen to a song and find your tension sub-siding just a little—down to, say, 6. This shows that this song may be a good candidate for your soothing play-list—it has made you feel somewhat more relaxed. Then do your second listen to it, matching your breathing to the pace of the music—having your body actually follow along with the tune, rhythm and pacing. Now suppose, after a minute or two, you really do feel relaxed—down to a 3, for example. Congratulations! You have found a song for your soothing playlist! Keep it and self-tune another soothing song.

Repeat this process with each of your first selection of songs—the ones you usually find soothing. Keep those that are really relaxing for you—that lower your tension level when you match your breathing to their pacing and rhythm. If, while listening, you notice anything bother-some or something that pokes at your tension, then set that song aside—it may be a perfectly fine one, but it does not belong in your soothing playlist. For example, some songs may have slow, quiet portions for a while, then speedier sections. Matching your breathing to those songs' overall pacing may lead you away from relaxation—even though the first section may make you feel peaceful and quiet, the next segment may pull you in a different direc-tion. While you may like a song a lot, if it is not soothing to you, it should not be in your soothing playlist.

As you assemble your soothing playlist, you will prob-ably notice that the best soothing songs are ones with consistent tempo and instrumentation—too many chang-es in speed, loudness or softness, or use of instruments will tend to pull you away from relaxation.

After you put together a soothing playlist with in-strumentals, consider adding vocals if there are ones you like. Follow the same self-tuning approach: first rate your pre-listening tension on the 1 to 9 scale; listen for a minute or so, then rate your tension again to determine if the song is soothing—*for you*; if so, listen again to the song, this time matching your breathing to the music, and again use the 1 to 9 scale to see if your tension level has dropped more. Vocal songs may be distracting by leading you to focus on the words, but vocals with which you are highly familiar, or ones in which the words are simple and repetitious—and sung in a warm, soothing manner—may work for you.

Remember that just because a song does not fit into your soothing playlist, that does not make it a bad song or one you should stop listening to. It just means that when you specifically want music that will soothe you, that particular song will probably be ineffective.

After you put together a soothing playlist, use the same self-tuning method to create a mood-boosting play-list. Choose several songs—instrumentals only at first—that perk you up or make you feel better when you "have the blues" because of the weather, a problem at work, per-sonal issues, or another cause. As before, find a cozy spot; wear loose, comfortable clothing; be sure you will not be disturbed for a while; and this time rate your "mood level" on a scale of 1 to 9, where 9 is "in a super-good mood" and 1 is "really feeling down and depressed."

Let's say you've had a frustrating day—a lot of little annoyances piled up—and you rate your mood a 3. After listening for a minute to the first mood-boosting song, perhaps you will find yourself feeling a little better—say, a 5. If so, the song is a candidate for the list. Now listen to it for a minute or so again, this time matching your breathing to the pace of the song while letting its rhythm, speed and instrumentation carry you along. Just let it flow through

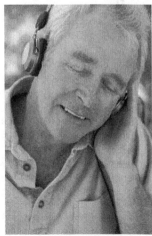

© Monkey Business - Fotolia.com

you as you match your breathing to it. After a minute or so, evaluate how you feel. Maybe you are feeling even a bit better now—say, a 6 or 7. Good! The song goes onto your feel-good playlist.

Repeat the whole process, from start to finish, with each candidate song, rejecting ones that create an up-and-down feeling—perhaps being peppy at first, then slowing down for a while and then speeding up again—keeping songs that make you feel energized with their rhythm. In this way, you will build a playlist to listen to when you need a mood boost.

Exercise Playlist

FOR A THIRD PLAYLIST, use self-tuning to get yourself moving—this is a playlist to use when exercising, whether running, working out at the gym, or doing crunches and free weights at home.

Listening to music during exercise can make the workout easier and more fun, by being a motivator so you exercise longer and more vigorously, while distracting you from negatives such as pain and fatigue. To enhance exercise, scientists have found that a song's tempo should be between 120 and 140 beats per minute, a pace that coincides with the range of most commercial dance music; many rock songs are near that range, too. If you exercise intensely, you may want songs at an even faster pace, around 150 beats per minute. But the good thing about self-tuning is that it does not require you to count beats or measure anything scientifically—you just have to *feel* the effects of the music *on you*.

So for a workout playlist, start as before in a relaxed, comfortable place, without interruptions, wearing loose clothing. This is your "resting state." For this playlist, you use the scale of 1 to 9 differently from the way you use it in the soothing and feel-good playlists. Here you start by deciding how rested you feel, with 1 being very laid-back and relaxed and 9 being highly energetic. In your resting state, you will probably start at a low number, perhaps a 3. Next, listen for about a minute to the first song that you expect to get you "pumped up." Rate on the scale how you feel after a minute—any more energetic? Maybe now you are at, say, a 5. Listen to the song again for another minute or so, this time matching your breathing to the song's pace and rhythm. You know that when you work out, you breathe faster and may even pant. That is the effect you want to get from the songs on this playlist—something that will enhance your body's natural response to exercise. After a minute or so of matching your breathing to the song, stop and rate how energized you feel. Maybe you are at a 7. Good! That song goes onto your workout playlist. Relax a bit to get back to your resting state, then test the next candidate song.

For the workout playlist, you may find that some songs with a slow start and speedup are effective at getting you going; or you may prefer ones that are fast-paced, maybe even intense, from the beginning to the end. Use whatever works for you!

In time, you may think of other kinds of playlists that you can create with self-tuning. If you have chronic pain, consider a "pain relief playlist"—find songs that take your mind off the pain and make you feel better. If you have seasonal allergies, think about making an "allergy playlist" with songs that relieve the feelings of congestion, itchy eyes and other symptoms. Playlists may not help tap the placebo response for every condition, but they can help in many ways and be used for many purposes. When you get the hang of self-tuning, you can make as many playlists as you want—and you may find them surprisingly effective at communicating with your cells and engaging their health-tropic tendencies.

Beyond the Playlist

PLAYLISTS ARE HIGHLY PERSONAL, but listening to music doesn't have to be a solo activity. Sitting with a friend and listening to music can be a bonding experience and a meaningful part of a relationship. You can even sing together. Or you might drum along with the beat—a longstanding tradition among indigenous people. When you drum, the rhythm becomes hypnotic and soothing, boosting the music's ability to get you out of your mind and into the moment—the now.

The mind-altering power of music is substantial, and engaging it is one of the best ways to harness the placebo effect. Explore many different types of music to determine what "turns you on," so to speak; what "lights your fire," what "moves" you and how. Music is entirely non-addictive and can be genuinely inspirational. Discover which pieces give *you* feelings of connection, warmth, relaxation, calm and uplift, and listen often!

The Pet Connection

YOU CAN ENHANCE the effectiveness of music by listening to it with your cat or dog. Like humans, dogs and cats are soothed and calmed by meditative music. You can give your pet a pleasurable experience while enhancing your own relaxation by petting your beloved animal friend while listening to music from your soothing playlist—or music that may not be on any of your playlists but that you simply enjoy. Scientists have found that petting a dog or cat lowers blood pressure. So when you listen to music *and* pet your furry friend, the pet calms down and bonds more closely with you—and you calm down as well, creating a positive feedback loop wherein the calming effects are extended and multiplied.

Music in Your Life

DIFFERENT TYPES OF MUSIC have very different effects, so you can use music for many purposes and make it a regular part of your day. If you regularly come home feeling stressed after work—because of a long commute, for example—use songs from your soothing playlist or feel-good playlist in the car and after you get home. If you are striving to make physical activity a regular part of your life, use your workout playlist regularly to get you "pumped up" and enthusiastic about movement and exercise.

Because music can pick you up or calm you down, sorting it into playlists gives you another way to adjust your mood and stay deeply "in tune" with your body—speeding up your breathing and heart rate when you need a pick-me-up, slowing your internal rhythm down when you need to relax, and so forth. Music affects us below the conscious level, bypassing the intellectual brain and putting us in touch with our beings all the way down to the level where our health-tropic cells work continuously to keep our bodies balanced and well. Use music—all kinds of music—throughout the day and in as many activities as you can, and you will find it a valuable tool for engaging your body's natural healing processes and making positive changes in your mood and your response to everyday frustrations and difficulties.

22

Enjoy Water

OUR BODIES ARE ABOUT TWO-THIRDS WATER—and the entire Earth is about two-thirds water, as well, being just one-third land. Water has a powerful draw on most of us and can be an excellent way to engage the relaxation response and, in so doing, "tell" our cells that we want them to maintain a health-tropic orientation and allow the placebo response to keep us well or restore us to health.

One of the wonderful things about water is that we can engage with it in so many different ways. Here are just a few examples—try them, and think of more on your own!

Take a Long, Hot Soak

DRAW A WARM BATH, and add a bit of bath oil to create a pleasing scent—choose something herbal to promote relaxation and stress reduction. Turn off bathroom lights, which are often bright and harsh, and light some candles. Play some music that you find relaxing quietly in the background. Then just soak, relaxing and meditating—or simply blanking your mind. The water around you "speaks" to the water in your body, promoting relaxation and stress reduction.

Indoor Water Fountain

THE PEACEFUL SOUND OF FLOWING WATER can be a great relaxer and stress reliever, and indoor fountains can be found at reasonable cost in a variety of gardening centers, department stores and specialty stores. For a more hand-son experience, you can even build your own fountain from a ceramic or metal container, a water pump, and a platform sponge from your local gardening shop. Find assembly instructions online—and decorate your fountain in whatever way you find most pleasant and relaxing. You can keep the fountain running all the time, or just when you know you tend to want extra stress reduction—perhaps in the evenings, between dinnertime and bedtime.

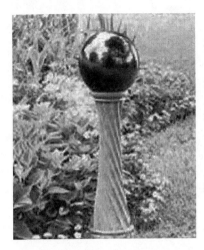

Gaze at a reflection, which carries your mind away. Watching fish in an aquarium can lower blood pressure and reduce stress. Anything floating in water is generally hypnotic. Some people find much relaxation in watching a gazing ball which seems to set the mind free in the multitude of reflections.

Open a Window on a Rainy Night

HERE IS A WAY to take advantage of weather that you might otherwise find depressing. Rain creates negative ions, which change the electrical charge in the air. Negative ions are refreshing. Plus there is something very soothing and relaxing about the sound and smell of soft, steady rain, even when it is cold rain in which you would not want to be out!. Simply open the window before you go to sleep and focus on the sounds of water outside— you will sleep better and awake refreshed.

Walk in the Rain

IT CAN BE EXCITING to venture outdoors during a rain-storm. In fact, if the rain is light, you may not even need an umbrella. A bit of light rain gently touching your skin can be quite relaxing and calming, putting your body in touch with all its internal water in a very direct tactile way. Even if the rain is a bit heavier and you need to carry an umbrella, being outdoors in a steady rain can be relaxing—although this works better if the rain is not *too* cold!

Take a Quick Dip

ANOTHER WAY in which water can effectively put you in touch with your cells and encourage their health-tropic behavior. After gentle exercise, or instead of it on some days, try doing a fast-paced swim in the pool. Swimming is great exercise, a wonderful way to stay in shape, and highly relaxing even as it gives your muscles a workout. Swimming gets your heart pumping and your muscles stretching, relieving stress and tension—and it promotes relaxation at the same time.

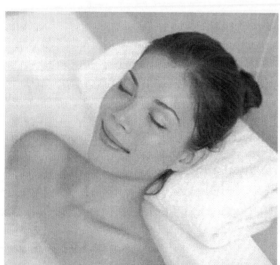

c Ariwasbi - Fotolia.com

There is something puri-fying, calm and clarifying about water—which in fact represents purity, clarity and calmness in Buddhist thinking. Because water is used to remove dirt, it is associates with cleanliness and the joy that we feel when we are clean, "rinsed free" of daily cares, concerns and worries. While immersing yourself in water—in any form, at any time— you can use the cleansing power of water to rid yourself of negative thoughts about your life and your health, allowing positive thinking to flow in instead. Feel the irritating events of the day wash away; imagine them flooded out of you and going down a drain, to disappear forever.

The purity symbolized by water can penetrate all parts of your mind and body, washing away ill will, unhappiness, ignorance and dissatisfaction—and providing a clean, pure basis for you to use when you start the next day. Engaging yourself regularly with water can help you stay focused on this sort of clarity and purity, which is just what your body needs symbolically to wash out—literally—disease and ill health.

23

Practice Qi Gong

WE ARE ENERGY BEINGS. Energy flows through our bodies. Like a kind of electricity, energy flows through our nerves. Red blood cells, which are infused with nourishment, flow through our blood vessels like a river of energy. Like microwaves and radio waves—which we cannot perceive but which we know are all around us—we have similar invisible energy waves in our body called *meridians,* along which there is a constant flow of *chi* or *qi*—pronounced "chee."

In Chinese medicine, chi is considered to be the life force. As a blood vessel can be narrowed or blocked by plaque and starve a muscle or organ, leading to a cascade of health problems, so too the chi that flows along meridians can be blocked, leading to health decline.

You may wonder at calling chi the life force. If not chi, then what? Where is the life force? If there is a life force and you are alive, it must be in your body, right? What makes your heart beat? The Chinese call the force that makes your heart beat chi. The chi energy flows through the entire body.

You can learn to manage and direct your chi. When you enhance your chi, you can send healing energy throughout your body, right down to your cells, which is where healing takes place—where you harness the placebo effect and bring about a return to wellness.

Before you can use your chi, however, you must experience it so that you can recognize it. This is easy to do within a couple of minutes, even if this is your first attempt.

Experience Your Chi

Stand in a relaxed position with your arms and hands hanging at your side.

Notice how your arms and hands feel hanging there. Study sensations in your arms and hands. Be aware of the heaviness of your arms and hands as they hang from your shoulders. Feel how gravity pulls on them as they hang down. Notice where the hands join the arm and how that point, the wrist, feels like a movable hinge. Feel the connection between wrist and arm—where they join—the looseness of the joining up to a point, then the tightness when you can move the wrist so far and no farther.

Bring your hands together in front of you and rub them vigorously, the way you would if you were out in the cold without gloves. Continue rubbing your hands for thirty seconds to a minute until you feel a strong sensation of warmth. Feel the warmth building as you rub. Feel the friction of palm against palm. Be aware of how one part of your skin feels when touching another part. Notice how your hands glide over each other, whether easily or roughly. Be aware of your skin texture and whether it is the same on both hands or different.

Let your hands fall easily to your side again and gently shake your hands and arms. Keep shaking them gently for 30 seconds or so. Feel gravity's pull on your hands. Notice the way your hands and arms move—how they feel almost like rubber as you shake them gently.

Then let your arms and hands hang loosely at your side again. Now notice the tingling sensations in your hands and fingertips, flowing in your arms. This tingling is your chi. Study how it feels. Close your eyes and focus on the tingling sensation, which is your life force. Notice how it flows. Be aware of the little pinpricks of sensation as your chi flows. Feel the chi move from place to place. Feel it ebb and flow as you focus on it.

The chi you activated by rubbing your hands and shaking your arms is circulating throughout your body, stimulating and nourishing your cells. You can reach into your body and communicate directly with your cells by activating and moving your chi—your life force, your healing energy.

Keep in mind that you are not a single entity—you are a community of individual living cells, a colony organism. It is through chi that you can reach into your body to interact with your family of cells. When you focus your mind on your chi energy, you are in the present moment, rather than the possibly troubling past or anxiety-provoking future. You begin to feel calmer because you are not thinking worrisome thoughts but are energizing yourself instead.

Once you feel your chi, you are ready to learn qi gong.

Practicing Qi Gong

QI GONG IS EASY TO LEARN and easy to practice. By doing the above "experiencing" exercise, you have already
begun to use your chi. It is that easy. The more you learn
and the more you practice, the more easily you can manage your chi to heal and revitalize yourself by engaging
your inner bio-community.

Qi gong doesn't require special equipment, clothing
or machines. It is something you can begin doing right
now, by yourself or with a friend—even right next to your
desk. Practicing for just a few minutes is refreshing.

Qi gong is related to other Eastern practices, such as
acupuncture, which uses needles to stimulate specific
points through which chi energy flows. Tai Chi, which is
another way of harnessing and using chi energy, promotes physical and mental
balance and calm, but takes   *Your chi flows faster and*
time and discipline to master.   *deeper when your mind*
Yoga brings feelings of sup-   *and body are relaxed.*
pleness, relaxation and peace,   —Lee Holden
but it also takes a while to be-
come proficient in it. All these
chi-related practices are beneficial, but qi gong is particularly easy and quick to learn.

Qi gong is reported to have a positive impact on pain,
especially that of arthritis, and to promote greater movement. People say they notice an increase in stamina
almost immediately after practicing qi gong. Qi gong is
also reported to reduce high blood pressure and soothe
stress.

The purpose of the ancient Chinese practices, whether qi gong, tai chi or yoga, is to circulate your chi flow so your body can heal itself naturally. Qi gong is an effortless practice, slow and graceful—there is nothing pushy or forceful about it. Results come surprisingly quickly as the chi energy circulates through damaged areas, triggering the healing process. Short sessions of 3 to 5 minutes a couple of times a day are good and can usually be squeezed into our hectic modern lives.

Lee Holder, a popular Qi gong master seen on public television and author of numerous Qi Gong DVD trainings, suggests developing your own rituals, say in the morning and in the evening, where you do a short qi gong practice. Swinging your body upon arising in the morning gets your energy moving around gently and quickly—faster than coffee, which must make its way through the digestive system. Qi gong helps you start off the day feeling well and filled with vitality. Doing your qi gong ritual for a few minutes again in the evening helps you wind down in preparation for restful sleep.

Qi gong is a full-body stimulation system of stretching, breathing, knocking various acupuncture points, and movement. Just a few minutes of qi gong exercises can leave you feeling refreshed and recharged, able to take on the world.

The Gates of Life

THERE IS A PRESSURE POINT on the lower back called Life Gates. In the following exercise, you hit your hand on that point, which stimulates blocked-up energy to break through and flow. Here's how.

Stand with your feet apart, about the width of your shoulders. Notice how you feel. Rate your level of tension on a scale of 1, for no tension, to 9, for extreme tension. How tense do you feel right now?

Let your body relax, with your arms hanging at your side, and slowly twist to one side all the way. Stop briefly. Then twist all the way to the other side. Twist from side to side fast enough that your arms swing and your hands swing out. Let them swing all the way until they are stopped by hitting your body—with one hand hitting in the middle of your lower back and the other in the middle of your abdomen. There are acupressure points at these points: the Life Gates.

After swinging and knocking for a few minutes, slowly let your body unwind until you are again standing still. Notice the sensations you feel: the loosening tension in your muscles, the weight pulling down your arms and hands as you slow down the swinging and knocking, the sensation of tingling in your arms and your back. All of this is your chi. Now rate your level of tension again, on the scale of 1 being very low tension and 9 being very high tension.

How does your tension level before swinging compare to the level after you swung around several times? If you are like most people, you probably noticed a drop in your tension level. If so, *you did this yourself,* and in only a few minutes, on your *first* practice. That is impressive.

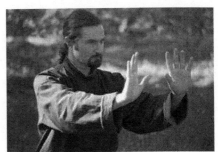

© furmananna - Fotolia.com

It is through this sort of process that you can learn to manage your chi and thereby manage your energy level and wellness.

Now close your eyes and simply focus on the feeling of your chi circulating. You have shown yourself that you can experience results with this method. Qi gong is amazingly simple and natural. People who practice qi gong routines regularly report feelings of wellness. Having more energy feels good, which is why energy drinks sell so well. We drink them to rev ourselves up with an infusion of an external stimulant, instead of learning how to stimulate our own natural energy from within.

Chi is like water. When stopped up it can become stagnant, but when flowing it has vitality.

Continuous stress, especially if coupled with inadequate rest, can damage the body's healing ability. The unique thing about qi gong is its paradoxical effect: feeling infused with energy and simultaneously relaxed. As you learn the various points and ways to stimulate them, you can give yourself a kind of body tune-up. As you work your chi you notice more vitality, purpose and health from the inside out—feeling good with only a few minutes of practice a day.

With simple stretches and movements, such as rolling your head and neck while breathing slowly and deeply, you can stretch the muscles in your neck to release chi, which then relieves tension from your neck and shoulders. With these simple techniques you manage and operate your bio-robot, keeping it limber and healthy.

We can hold energy as tension or we can hold energy as flow. Flow feels better. Qi gong helps us learn to manage the polarity of tension and flow. Tension is tightness, restriction and stagnation and leads to disease and decline; energy-circulating flow creates a powerful integral state. Here are some ways to improve flow of your healing chi.

Shaking

STAND AGAIN IN A RELAXED MANNER with your feet about shoulder width apart, allowing your arms to hang loosely at your side. As before, take a quick survey of your feelings and sensations, again rating your level of tension on a scale with 1 being low and 9 being very high tension.

Now imagine that your arms, down through your wrists and into your hands, are like rubber. Slowly shake your rubber-like hands and arms. Just keep shaking your arms and hands while reminding yourself that they are pliable and flexible, like rubber. This shakes out stress and pressure.

Bouncing

WHILE CONTINUING TO SHAKE, add an easy bounce so that you are shaking and bouncing, like a rag doll in a cartoon. This creates a pump-like action that gets fluids flowing up and down your spine—literally flowing.

Bobbing Head

IMAGINE THAT YOUR HEAD is like one of those bobble-head dolls that people put on the dashboard of their cars. As you continue to shake and bounce, let your head bounce like the dashboard doll's head.

When you feel like it, just slow your shaking and bouncing to come to an easy stop. Stand for a few seconds while again noticing how you feel. Observe the inward sensations and energy flowing inside you—your chi, your life force energy. Again, rate your tension level on the 1 to 9 scale and compare your "after" feelings to those before you tried the exercise.

In the Present

TO HARNESS CHI most effectively, drop into the present moment. Try this now. Feel the air going through your fingers—the sensation of movement of air, the sensitivity of your fingertips, the way the air and your body interact. Sense and notice the feel of your clothes, feel the air around you, feel the brush of hair on your neck. How lightly or heavily do your clothes lie on your skin? How does your skin feel when touching the fabric? How does the air moving past you feel? Does your hair tickle your skin, rub it, lie on it lightly or heavily? *Feel* instead of think.

In qi gong, there are two energies, one energy for the mind and one energy for the body. The body energy is the fuel—think of breathing in to fill your fuel tank. The second energy involves having a clear intention—having a direction, an intention. When you think of your intention while breathing in you will feel more powerful and more focused. Learn to turn your awareness inward to feel your chi energy, which also brings you into the moment, helping you let go of the past and avoid worries about the future.

Rapid Mood Change

BY UNDERSTANDING CHI and using qi gong, you can change your mood quickly by changing your posture and your expressions. For example, when you feel depressed, you will tend to hunch your shoulders over and hang your head, which causes shallow breathing that diminishes chi and brings on depression. You can change your feelings and mood quickly by raising your eyebrows and smiling. By changing your expression and posture, you change your chi flow—which lifts your mood. This is you managing your bio-robot with simple movements.

Another example: by standing up straight and throwing your shoulders back, you will find it easier to breathe in deeply—the posture opens you up and releases your chi so it flows more freely. Similarly, when feeling sad, we tend to frown, letting our head droop while looking down—which constricts chi flow. By raising your eyebrows, you lift up your face and head. Then with smiling you lift up your face even more and your chi flows freely—which you can feel quickly.

Use the movements of qi gong every day, several times a day, to keep you in touch with the physical sensations of your body and the internal feelings of chi flow. Because qi gong is so easy to learn and so simple to do, you can practice it just about anywhere, and it takes only a small amount of time. Practicing qi gong movements a few times a day will enhance your energy flow to stimulate your cells, again and again, letting them know that you want them to engage in health-tropic behavior to keep you well and prevent disease and discomfort from taking over your body. Qi gong and the chi flow that it manages are powerful but simple ways of engaging the placebo effect—of informing your body again and again that you want to be well and remain well.

24

Take a Sauna

WHEN IT COMES TO making a significant change in our bodies' environment to "wake up" our cells, few approaches beat that of spending time in a sauna. A sauna's dry heat, which can get as high as 185 degrees Fahrenheit, has profound and nearly immediate effects on the body. Skin temperature soars to about 104 degrees Fahrenheit within minutes. The average person will pour out a pint of sweat during a short stint in a sauna. In a sauna, your pulse rate jumps by 30% or more, allowing your heart to nearly double the amount of blood it pumps each minute. Most of the extra blood flow is directed to the skin—in fact, your body actually shunts blood away from internal organs. Blood pressure, though, is unpredictable, rising in some people but falling in others.

"All in all, saunas appear safe for the body, but there is little evidence that they have health benefits above and beyond relaxation and a feeling of well-being," says Harvey B. Simon, M.D., editor-in-chief of *Harvard Men's Health Watch*. But to engage the placebo effect—which itself provides significant health benefits—relaxation and a feeling of well-being are exactly what we want. So saunas are certainly worth considering—although if you are a heart patient, be sure to check with your doctor before taking a sauna.

Known Benefits

THE RELAXATION BENEFITS of saunas are undoubted. They relieve many symptoms of stress, relaxing muscles and soothing aches and pains in muscles and joints. The high heat of saunas causes the body to release endorphins, our natural pain-relieving hormones, resulting in a mild, enjoyable tranquilizing effect that can soothe people with arthritis as well as athletes after an intense workout. The increased blood flow resulting from a sauna's causing blood vessels to dilate helps speed the body's natural healing processes, helping cuts and bruises get better more quickly, relieving muscle tension and flushing out lactic acid and other post-workout toxins.

The heat of a sauna causes sweating, of course. However, this is not ordinary sweating but *deep sweating*, which can help reduce our bodies' levels of such contaminants as lead, copper, zinc, nickel and mercury. The sweat rinses bacteria out of the epidermal layer and sweat ducts, cleansing our pores and giving our skin a softer appearance. Deep sweating helps plump up tiny wrinkles and maintain our skin's collagen structure, reducing sagging.

What the Heat Does

THE HEAT OF A SAUNA induces deeper sleep, so your body is better able to repair any damage incurred during the day and help you start the next day feeling fresh. Furthermore, although heart patients must use saunas with care because of a sauna's effect on the cardiovascular system, there is evidence that sauna use can actually strengthen the heart: your heart rate goes from its usual 60 to 70 beats per minute to 110 to 120 beats, which means cardiac output increases—and this can be particularly helpful for people with congestive heart failure, whose hearts are unable to pump blood efficiently. Sitting in a sauna is equivalent to doing mild exercise—your cardiovascular system reacts the same way. And that means, among other things, that using a sauna burns calories, since higher cardiovascular activity prompts the body to convert more calories to energy. This is one very direct way in which sauna use influences our non-conscious communication with our cells.

There are other direct benefits of saunas, too. They can relieve sinus congestion from colds or allergies, especially when a sauna—which normally provides dry heat—is used with steam, which breaks up that congested feeling.

Precautions

BECAUSE THE SAUNA is so different from what we experience in everyday life, there are some precautions to follow if you want to try it. Avoid alcohol and any medications that may impair sweating and produce overheating before and after your sauna. Stay in for no more than 15 to 20 minutes, then cool down gradually afterwards. Drink two to four glasses of cool water after each sauna. And do not take a sauna when you are ill—in fact, if you feel unwell during your sauna, head for the door.

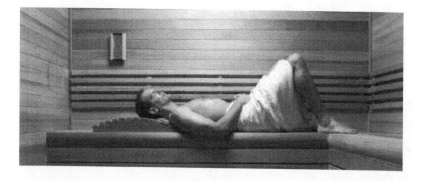

It is worth mentioning that saunas are being studied as possibly beneficial for a number of diseases—in addition to their ability to put us into a relaxed state that engages the health-tropic inclinations of our cells. For at least some people, saunas have proved directly helpful in treating chronic fatigue, mild depression, rheumatoid arthritis, musculoskeletal pain and various skin conditions. If you have any of these conditions, ask your doctor whether you should consider taking a sauna for relief—you may start to feel better almost immediately.

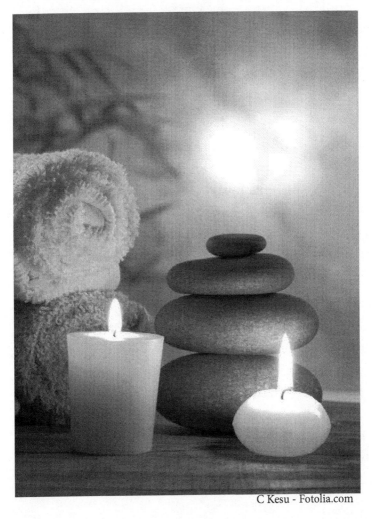

C Kesu - Fotolia.com

25

Use Tapping

OUR ABILITY TO TAP INTO THE PLACEBO EFFECt has increased interest in systems used for centuries—even millennia—that have in the past been rejected by traditional disease-focused Western medicine. Studies of systems such as acupuncture have shown an underlying scientific basis for healing claims that were long rejected as being based on fantasy—as acupuncture is based on the Chinese concept of qi or energy flow, a notion rejected by Western medicine.

As the limitations of treating problems with pills to kill pain, suppress anxiety and make it possible to sleep at night have become clearer, more people have turned to non-invasive approaches to health maintenance and restoration—and a variety of new ones have sprung up, being based on old non-Western approaches and claiming to adapt them to the modern world.

One of those is *tapping*. This is a simple-to-master system whose proponents claim it provides relief from chronic pain, emotional problems, disorders, addictions, phobias, post-traumatic stress, and physical diseases. Tapping is rooted in the healing concepts that have been in practice in Asian medicine for over 4,000 years, and is related to acupuncture and acupressure. It uses the body's *energy meridian points*, which you stimulate yourself by tapping them with your fingertips. Think of it as a form of acupuncture without needles and without an acupuncturist being involved.

The Basics

TAPPING PROPONENTS say your health must be approached holistically, with an understanding that we experience negative emotions through a disruption in the body's energy flow—physical pain and disease are intertwined with negative emotions. Thus, health problems create a kind of vicious cycle in which physical symptoms trigger emotional distress, and emotional problems manifest through physical symptoms. Using tapping to engage the body's self-healing process—the placebo effect, although that is not what tapping advocates call it—breaks the cycle and allows health to flow.

Like everything in the universe, the body is composed of energy. In the Asian view of healing, when you restore energy balance, negative emotions and physical symptoms that stemmed from the energy disruption are released. Tapping is said to restore the body's energy balance and release negative emotions.

Unlike placebo-effect approaches that encourage positive thoughts and optimism, in tapping you focus on the negative emotion—such as a fear or anxiety, a bad memory, or an unresolved problem. While keeping your attention on the negative emotion, you tap 5-7 times with your fingertips on each of a series of meridian points. It is believed that tapping on the meridian points, while concentrating on accepting and resolving the troublesome emotional issue, accesses the body's energy to restore it to balance.

There are many Web sites and online videos that show what tapping is and how it works—and it is easy to learn. So you can try it yourself without difficulty— just search for the term and check the written and video materials. If a particular demonstration or written explanation seems confusing, or you simply do not like it, just move on to the next—there are plenty of them, and you will soon find ones that explain tapping in ways with which you are comfortable.

Meridians

THE FOUNDATION OF TAPPING is the notion that energy circulates through your body along a network of channels and that you can tap into this energy at points along the system. The concept is rooted in traditional Chinese medicine. The energy is called qi or ch'i and pronounced "chee." Some 3000 to 4000 years ago, the Chinese discovered 100 meridian points, which when stimulated could heal. This is the origin of acupuncture, which uses very thin needles to stimulate those points. Tapping simply uses finger taps instead of needles—which means you can tap anywhere, anytime, without any special equipment.

Acupuncture practitioners, on the other hand, must memorize hundreds of meridian points along the body; the knowledge and training take years to master. So it is easy to see why proponents advocate tapping: it is simple, painless, free, and requires nothing more than your own fingertips. And if you believe it will work—as is the case with other methods of engaging the placebo effect— then it may bring you benefits.

There is an underlying philosophy supported by advocates of tapping, which is that the process puts the power to heal yourself into your hand—your fingertips, to be specific. You are in charge of your own health and healing.

Skepticism

TAPPING HAS BEEN MET WITH SKEPTICISM in the world of Western medicine, with traditional doctors and psychologists being quick to dismiss it because there are no controlled clinical trials or research studies showing that it has any effect whatsoever. However, this ignores the considerable anecdotal evidence from practitioners and people who have experienced it—and the power of the placebo effect in general.

Recent studies of the placebo effect have shown that it produces real, lasting breakthroughs and significantly improves or sometimes even eliminates conditions that hospital treatments, medication and years of psychotherapy often fail to handle adequately. To the extent that tapping engages the placebo effect, it can certainly have some benefit for some people—and it costs nothing to try it and requires little time to learn it.

Studies done at Harvard Medical School found that the brain's stress and fear response, which is controlled by the amygdala—an almond-shaped part of the brain—can be reduced by stimulating the meridian points. This research used acupuncture. Tapping advocates say stimulating the points with pressure works just as well. Certain tapping proponents claim significant anecdotal success with the technique. For example, Dawson Church, Ph.D., who leads seminars on tapping using the term Emotional Freedom Techniques (EFT) for the training, says people's levels of cortisol—a stress hormone—dropped 24% after a one-hour tapping session he supervised. An author of numerous books on health and spirituality, Church says that he used tapping on war veterans suffering from post-traumatic stress disorder (PTSD)—and that it produced an average 63% decrease in PTSD symptoms after six sessions.

So far scientists have not replicated these results, which may be related to conventional psychological techniques employed by tapping practitioners along with the tapping itself—without evidence that any improvements were connected to body-energy mechanisms. But it is not necessary to become involved in the scientific claims and counterclaims about tapping in order to try it for yourself—no costly seminar or supervising practitioner is needed, since tapping is so easy to learn. The whole point of the placebo effect is to harness the body's own natural healing powers to boost your health, and if you find that tapping does this for you, you will have discovered an easy, inexpensive method of helping your body make itself feel better. Proponents say thousands of people use it with benefits.

Try It Yourself

ONE GOOD WAY to decide whether tapping will engage your body's placebo effect is by simply following along with the online demonstration videos and noticing how it feels to you. Another good way is to create your own exercise, using tapping techniques.

Try this now. Identify a person or situation that you find really frustrating. It may be at home or work, or could involve a friend whose behavior has been getting to you. Pick something that has been on your mind lately.

Focus on your frustration about this situation. Close your eyes and concentrate on the situation and how frustrated it makes you feel. Notice sensations in your body that seem connected to this frustration, such as tightness in your jaw or neck, or a clenching of your stomach.

Rate the intensity of your frustration on a scale of 1 to 9, with 1 being no frustration and 9 being extremely frustrated.

Write a Frustration Focus Statement describing how you feel—and then asserting your power over the feeling. For example: *"Even though I feel this frustration in my stomach, I deeply and completely accept myself."*

The key is to focus on and acknowledge the frustration, tell yourself just how it is affecting you physically, and then create a self-affirmation that you are not going to let the frustration damage your health or dominate your thinking.

Say your *Frustration Focus Statement* three times while you continuously tap on the first accu-point, which is the karate-chop point on the hand— the soft fleshy part of your hand, located between your wrist and pinky

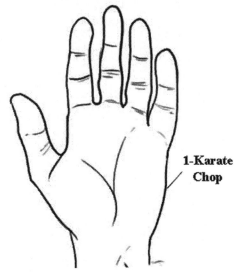

1-Karate Chop

finger. If you are right-handed, tap lightly on the karate chop of your left hand with the tips of the pointer, middle and ring fingers of your right hand. Tap with a constant beat (one tap per second or a bit faster) while saying your Frustration Focus statement three times. It is important to really mean it when you say that you accept yourself even though you have the negative feelings.

If you are right-handed, use the body points on the right side; use the left side points if you are left-handed. Reach over to the other side of the body for the underarm point—that is, if you are right-handed, reach across to the underarm spot on your left side.

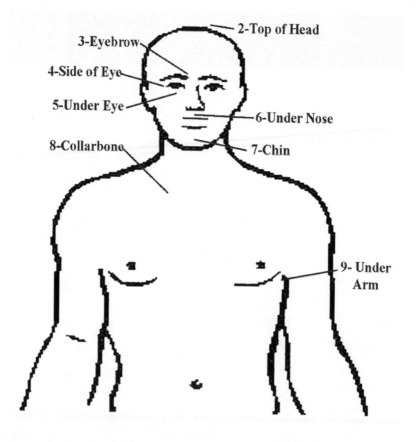

As you tap on the series of body points, use an abbreviated statement that has only two of the words, such as "this frustration." Say the shortened statement once while gently and continuously tapping five to seven times on each of the body points (points 2 to 9 in the diagram).

Repeat this sequence as you tap on each point in the diagram. Tap on the top of your head while saying "this frustration." Then tap on the eyebrow bone where it meets your nose while saying "this frustration." Next, tap on the bone at the far side of your eye while saying "this frustration." The next point is tapping on the bone right under the middle of your eye, while saying "this frustration." Then tap under your nose while saying, "this frustration." Then tap on your chin while saying "this frustration." The next point to tap is on the collarbone— again, while saying "this frustration." Lastly, tap the underarm point while saying "this frustration."

Take a slow, deep breath when you finish this sequence, and gently stretch your neck and roll your shoulders.

Focus again on the location in your body where you felt the frustration. Rate the intensity of your frustration using the same scale of 1 to 9, with 1 being no or very low frustration and 9 being extremely frustrated. If the ending intensity level is higher than 5, repeat the sequence. Change your Frustration Focus statement slightly, for example to: "Even though I *still* feel this frustration in my stomach, I deeply and completely accept myself" and change the shortened statement to: "This *remaining* frustration."

More Statements

HERE are some additional sample Frustration Focus Statements:

> "Even though I feel this anxious knot in my stomach, I deeply and completely accept myself."

> "Even though I feel angry because my friend ignored me, I deeply and completely accept myself."

> "Even though I feel mad at myself for making a mistake, I deeply and completely accept myself."

> "Even though I feel this sharp pain in my lower back, I deeply and completely accept myself."

> "Even though I feel jealous of my friend's success, I deeply and completely accept myself."

> "Even though I have this pounding headache, I deeply and completely accept myself."

The more specifically you can state your physical, emotional or mental discomfort or pain, the more powerful the statement will be in helping you focus on releasing bound-up emotion and pain.

Discussion

WHAT EMOTIONS CAME UP while you did the tapping? What energy shifts did you notice in your body, such as in your stomach, chest or throat? What change in physical sensations did you experience—increase, decrease or movement? What thoughts came up while tapping? Consider another tapping session, using these thoughts, if they are negative or distressing.

Tapping is not a cure-all and will not work for everybody. Like other techniques for engaging the placebo response, it requires a strong belief that it will work—or it will not. One great thing about tapping is that it is simple to learn and does not require any guide, helper or practitioner. You can learn it in privacy, try it on your own, and decide for yourself whether it has any validity for you. If it does not, you can simply abandon it and move on to other methods of engaging the placebo effect.

Index

Authors

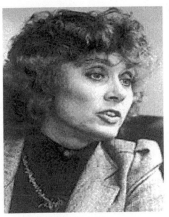

Beverly A. Potter, Ph.D, (Docpotter) received her doctorate in counseling psychology from Stanford University and her masters in vocational rehabilitation counseling from San Francisco State University. She is a self-help author noted for challenging rules and thinking of issues from a fresh perspective. Her work blends philosophies of humanistic psychology, social learning theory and Eastern philosophies to create an inspiring and original approach to handling the many difficulties encountered today. Beverly provides keynote speeches and training. Her offices are in Oakland, California. (www.docpotter.com)

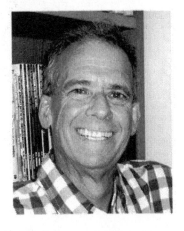

Mark James Estren, Ph.D, received his doctorates in psychology and in English from University of Buffalo and his master's degree in journalism from Columbia University. He is a Pulitzer-winning journalist who has held top-level positions at several newspapers and TV news organizations for over 30 years, including *The Washington Post, Miami Herald, Philadelphia Inquirer, CBS* and *ABC News* and other news media. He was one of *Fortune* magazine's "People to Watch." Early in his career, Mark ran *Financial News Network* and was the editor of *High Technology Business* magazine. Mark's offices are in Ft. Myers, Florida. (www.markjestren.com)